The Coɪ
of Aphe

Eisei Noiri
Norio Hanafusa
Editors

The Concise Manual of Apheresis Therapy

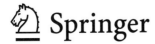 Springer

Editors

Eisei Noiri
Department of Hemodialysis
 & Apheresis
The University of Tokyo
 Hospital
Bunkyo-ku, Tokyo, Japan

Norio Hanafusa
Department of Hemodialysis
 & Apheresis
The University of Tokyo
 Hospital
Bunkyo-ku, Tokyo, Japan

ISBN 978-4-431-54411-1   ISBN 978-4-431-54412-8 (eBook)
DOI 10.1007/978-4-431-54412-8
Springer Tokyo Heidelberg New York Dordrecht London

Library of Congress Control Number: 2013951138

This English translation is based on the Japanese original Apheresis Ryoho Pocket Manual by Eisei Noiri and Norio Hanafusa (eds) © 2012 Ishiyaku Publishers, Inc.

Printed on acid-free paper

Springer is part of Springer Science+Business Media (www.springer.com)

Preface

The word "apheresis" which is of Greek origin, means "taking away" in English. Apheresis is a mode of therapy specifying a certain target and removing it from the body. Given the target of immunoglobulin, antibodies, or virus particles, apheresis constitutes a blood purification therapy that is presumably antithetical to hemodialysis, which is the most popular blood purification therapy worldwide. Although each removes a blood component, hemodialysis is often prescribed to rid the body of uremic toxins, even though the actual uremic toxin targets have not been clarified to date. The prescription of apheresis must nearly always include initial consideration of the characteristics of the pathogenetic target to enable its elimination through distribution, filtration, and adsorption or centrifugation. Apheresis is becoming a therapy that is not only limited to methods of withdrawal for pathogenic compounds. It is now applicable for use as a supplemental approach, per contra, for defective components underlying certain diseases. Therefore, it is no exaggeration to say that blood purification therapies are aiming at apheresis as the ultimate mode of therapy. Whenever the recent advances in life science reveal a particular causative target for a certain disease, apheresis can be used to eliminate it and save lives. Today, apheresis has become an indispensable choice of therapy in flagship hospitals. Apheresis in Japan has developed uniquely by virtue of the state-of-the-art textile industry underlying its processes and components. Double-filtration plasma pheresis (DFPP), low-density lipoprotein (LDL)-apheresis, and granulocyte apheresis (GCAP) deserve special notice because of their efficient modalities of Japanese origin.

However, the essence of this book is its complete sharing of common knowledge, making it a must-have whenever caring for patients using apheresis.

"Knowledge exists to be imparted."

Ralph Waldo Emerson

I earnestly hope that this concise book will facilitate and encourage the practice of apheresis all over the world.

Bunkyo-ku, Tokyo, Japan   Eisei Noiri

Contents

x   Contents

Part IV   Autoimmune Disorders

List of Notes

- Removal by Biologically Specific Reactions
- Buffy Coat
- Combination of PE with HD and Hemodiafiltration
- Outcome from PDF/the MELD Score
- Substances Adsorbed with Hemoperfusion
- Effectiveness of LCAP for Rheumatoid Arthritis
- Estimation of Plasma Volume
- Catheter Development
- Heparin-Induced Thrombocytopenia
- Reduction of FXIII Levels During Apheresis Therapies
- Apheresis for Isaac's Syndrome
- Apheresis for N-Methyl-D-Aspartate Receptor (NMDAR) Encephalitis
- Apheresis for Miller–Fischer Syndrome
- Chronic Inflammatory Demyelinating Polyneuropathy Associated with Monoclonal Gammopathy of Undetermined Significance
- Apheresis for Neuromyelitis Optica
- Recurrence of FSGS After Kidney Transplantation
- The Effect of Cytapheresis on MPO-ANCA Associated Vasculitis
- Prevention of Neonatal Conduction Failure by IAPP
- Anti-PP1Pk Antibody/Administration of Anti-D Immunoglobulin (RHIG) into Non-immunized Women/ Anti-phospholipid Antibody Syndrome
- Enlargement of Indications for LDL Apheresis
- PMX-DHP May Have Other Effects Beyond Endotoxin Absorption
- Albumin Dialysis

- Pathogenesis of TTP/TMA
- The Future of the Apheresis for Removal of Leukocytes
- MARS (Molecular Adsorbent Recirculating System, MARS®)
- ABO-Incompatible Transplantation

Abbreviations

A

ABI	Ankle brachial index
ACD	Acid citrate dextrose fluid
ACEI	Angiotensin converting enzyme inhibitor
AchR	Acetylcholine receptor
ACR	American College of Rheumatology
ACT	Activated coagulation time/activated clotting time
ADAMTS-13	A disintegrin and metalloproteinase with thrombospondin type 1 motifs 13
ADL	Activities of daily living
AIP	Acute interstitial pneumonia
AKI	Acute kidney injury
ALI/ARDS	Acute lung injury/acute respiratory distress syndrome
allo-PBSCH	Allo-peripheral blood stem cell harvest (collection)
ALS	Artificial liver support
ANCA	Anti-neutrophil cytoplasmic antibody
APS	Antiphospholipid syndrome
APTT	Activated partial thromboplastin time
AQP4	Aquaporin 4
ARB	Angiotensin II receptor blocker
ASO	Arteriosclerosis obliterans
AT-III	Antithrombin-III
auto-PBSCH	Auto-peripheral blood stem cell harvest (collection)

B

BMT	Bone marrow transplantation
BP	Bullous pemphigoid

| BP-180 Ab | Anti BP-180 antibody |
| BP-230 Ab | Anti BP-230 antibody |

C

CAPS	Catastrophic APS
CART	Cell-free and concentrated ascites re-infusion therapy
CD	Crohn's disease
CDAI	Chrohn's disease activity index
CDC	Complement dependent cytotoxicity
CF	Circulating factors
CHD	Continuous hemodialysis
CHDF	Continuous hemodiafiltration
CHF	Continuous hemofiltration
CIDP	Chronic inflammatory demyelinating polyneuropathy
CL	Cardiolipin
CMV	Cytomegalovirus
CPE	Continuous plasma exchange
CPMS	Chronic progressive MS
CRP	C-reactive protein
CRRT	Continuous renal replacement therapy
CY	Cyclophosphamide
CyA	Cyclosporin A

D

DAS	Disease activity score
DFPP	Double filtration plasmapheresis
DHP	Direct hemoperfusion
DIC	Disseminated intravascular coagulation
DIHS	Drug-induced hypersensitivity syndrome
DMARDs	Disease modifying anti-rheumatic drugs
DMSO	Dimethylsulfoxide
Dsg	Desmoglein
Dsg-1 Ab	Anti desmoglein-1 antibody
Dsg-3 Ab	Anti desmoglein-3 antibody

E

EAA	Endotoxin activity assay
EBA	Epidermolysis bullosa acquisita
EOG	Ethylene oxide gas
ESR	Erythrocyte sedimentation rate
EUPHAS	Early use of polymyxin B hemoperfusion in abdominal septic shock
EUVAS	European Vasculitis Study Group

F

FXIII	factor XIII
FCXM	Flow cytometric crossmatch
FFA	Free fatty acid
FFP	Fresh frozen plasma
FH	Familial hypercholesterolemia
FSGS	Focal segmental glomerulosclerosis

G

Gb3	Globotriaosylceramide
GBM	Glomerular basement membrane
GBS	Guillain–Barré syndrome
GCAP	Granulocytapheresis
G-CSF	Granulocyte-colony stimulating factor
GVHD	Graft versus host disease

H

HA	Hemoadsorption
HAM	HTLV-1-associated myelopathy
HBV	Hepatitis B virus
HCV	Hepatitis C virus
HD	Hemodialysis
HDF	Hemodiafiltration
HES	Hydroxyethyl starch
HF	Hemofiltration
HIT	Heparin induced thrombocytopenia
HLA	Human leukocyte antigens

HMGB-1	High mobility group B-1
HP	Hemoperfusion
HPC	Hematopoietic progenitor cell
HPT	Hepaplastin test
HSP	Henoch–Schönlein purpura
HUS	Hemolytic uremic syndrome

I

IAPP	Immunoadsorption plasma-pheresis
IBD	Inflammatory bowel diseases
IDL	Intermediate density lipoprotein
IFN	Interferon therapy
	IFN-gInterferon-g
IgA	Immunoglobulin A
IgG	Immunoglobulin G
IgM	Immunoglobulin M
IL	Interleukin
IPF	Idiopathic pulmonary fibrosis
IRB	Institutional review board
ITP	Idiopathic thrombocytopenic purpura
IVCY	Intravenous cyclophosphamide
IVIG	Intravenous immunoglobulin

L

LCAP	Leukocytapheresis
LDH	Lactate dehydrogenase
LDL	Low density lipoprotein
LDL-C	Low density lipoprotein cholesterol
LEMS	Lambert–Eaton myasthenic syndrome
LMWH	Low molecular weight heparin
LOHF	Late onset hepatic failure

M

MARS	Molecular Adsorbents Recirculation System
MBP	Myelin basic protein
MEPEX	Methylprednisolone versus plasma exchange

	(MEPEX) trial
MG	Myasthenia gravis
MGUS	Monoclonal gammopathy of undetermined significance
MMP	Mucous membrane pemphigoid
MMP-3	Matrix metalloproteinase-3
MOF	Multiple organ failure
MOG	Myelin oligodendrocyte glycoprotein
MPO-ANCA	Myeloperoxidase anti-neutrophil cytoplasmic antibody, P-ANCA
MRA	Malignant rheumatoid arthritis
MS	Multiple sclerosis
MuSK	Muscle-specific receptor tyrosine kinase

N

NKT	Natural killer T (NKT) cell
NM	Nafamostat mesilate
NMO	Neuromyelitis optica
NS	Nephrotic syndrome
NSAIDs	Nonsteroidal anti-inflammatory drugs

P

PA	Plasma adsorption
PAD	Peripheral arterial disease
PAN	Polyacrylonitrile
PBSCT	Peripheral blood stem cell transplantation
PE	Plasma exchange
PF	Pemphigus foliaceus
PMX	Toraymixin
PMX-DHP	Polymyxin-B immobilized column direct hemoperfusion
POC	Point-of-care
POLARIS	Prospective observational survey on the long-term effects of the LDL-apheresis on the drug resistant nephrotic syndrome
poly-HEMA	Poly-hydroxyethyl-methacrylate

PR3-ANCA	Proteinase 3-anti-neutrophil cytoplasmic antibody, C-ANCA
PSL	Prednisolone
PT	Prothrombin time
PV	Plasma volume
PV	Pemphigus vulgaris

Q

| QOL | Quality of life |

R

RA	Rheumatoid arthritis
RBC	Red blood cell, erythrocyte
RCT	Randomized controlled trial
RF	Rheumatoid factor
RHIG	Human anti-d immunoglobulin
RPGN	Rapidly progressive glomerulonephritis
RRMS	Relapsing-remitting MS

S

SC	Sieving coefficient
sFLC	Serum free light chains
SIRS	Systemic inflammatory response syndrome
SJS	Stevens–Johnson syndrome
SLE	Systemic lupus erythematosus
SPMS	Secondary progressive MS
SPP	Skin perfusion pressure
sTNFR	Soluble TNF receptor
SVR	Sustained virological response
SVRI	Systemic vascular resistance index

T

TEN	Toxic epidermal necrolysis
TG	Triglyceride
TIPS	Transjugular intrahepatic portosystemic shunt

TLR	Toll-like receptor
TMA	Thrombotic microangiopathy
TMP	Transmembrane pressure
	TNF-aTumor necrosis factor-a
TTP	Thrombotic thrombocytopenic purpura

U

UC	Ulcerative colitis
UFH	Unfractionated heparin

V

Vd	Volume of distribution
VGCC	Voltage-sensitive Ca2+ channel
VLDL	Very low-density lipoprotein
VRAD	Virus removal and eradication by DFPP
vWF	von Willebrand factor

W

WBC	White blood cells

Part I
Principles and Technologies

Chapter 1
Theoretical Background of Apheresis Therapy

Norio Hanafusa

Main Points

What Is Apheresis?
- Apheresis is a process used to separate and remove pathogenic substances within the blood.
- Plasma exchange is employed to supplement coagulation factors in patients with liver failure or thrombotic microangiopathy.

Properties of Therapies Relating to Removal of Pathogenic Substances.
- Most apheresis therapies require supplementation with blood-derived products. Mechanisms that enhance selectivity and specificity, including diffusion, filtration, adsorption, and centrifugation are used to reduce the volume of blood product supplementation.

N. Hanafusa (✉)
Department of Hemodialysis & Apheresis, University Hospital,
The University of Tokyo, 7-3-1 Hongo, Bunkyo-ku, Tokyo 113-8655, Japan
hanafusa-tky@umin.ac.jp

E. Noiri and N. Hanafusa (eds.), *The Concise Manual of Apheresis Therapy,* DOI 10.1007/978-4-431-54412-8_1, © Springer Japan 2014

Properties of Removed Substances.
- The efficacy of apheresis is determined by the relationship between the therapeutic method and properties of the target substance. The latter includes molecular weight, distribution volume, compartment, production rate (half-life), electric charge, hydrophilic or hydrophobic properties, and specific gravity.

1.1 What Is Apheresis?

1.1.1 Introduction

The word "apheresis" is derived from the ancient Greek word for "separation." Apheresis is a therapeutic process in which blood is drawn from the body, pathogenic substances are removed from the blood, and the blood is returned to the body.

The scope of apheresis is outlined in Table 1.1. Many diseases are potential targets for treatment with apheresis. The diseases that can be reimbursed for apheresis therapy by the Japanese government are listed in the last section of this book. These diseases include autoimmune disease, kidney disease, liver disease, gastrointestinal tract disorders, and hematologic disorders.

1.1.2 Elimination of Substances During Apheresis

The target diseases for apheresis are diverse in terms of both clinical efficacy and the pathogenic substances to be removed. It is important to determine the quantity of the substance eliminated during each apheresis session. The efficacy of substance removal from the blood is determined by two factors: specifications of the apheresis devices used and physical and chemical properties of the target molecules.

Each disease has a specific pathogenic target substance. The apheresis modality is determined from the nature of the

TABLE 1.1 Therapeutic modalities and their target substances

Therapeutic modality	Detailed modalities	Pathogenic substances to be removed
Plasmapheresis	Simple plasma exchange	Auto-antibodies
	Double filtration plasmapheresis	LDL cholesterol
		M proteins
		Toxins or wastes excreted by the liver
		Immune complex
		Hepatitis C virus (large amount of plasma infusion)
Cytapheresis	Leukocytapheresis	Leukocytes
	Granulocyte and monocyte apheresis	Granulocytes, monocytes
Direct hemoperfusion	β_2 microglobulin adsorption	$\beta_2$microglobulin, cytokines
	Activated charcoal	Toxins, drugs
	Polymyxin B immobilized column	Endotoxin, other pathogenic substances

target substance and treatment specifications. These points are discussed in the next chapter.

1.1.3 Supplementation of Substances by Apheresis

The original objective of apheresis was the removal of pathogenic substances. However, beneficial substances can also be replenished by plasma exchange. When replenishing coagulation factors, it is necessary to infuse a large quantity of fresh frozen plasma (FFP). Theoretically, FFP measuring as much as half of the patient's plasma volume is required to increase the concentration of coagulation factors by 50 %. For example, approximately 1.4 L of FFP are needed for a patient with a body weight of 60 kg and hematocrit of 35 %. A number of adverse events, including volume overload, can occur with frequent FFP infusions.

With apheresis, greater quantities of FFP can be infused through plasma exchange without volume overload, because the procedure removes an equal amount of plasma before infusion. The discarded plasma contains a smaller volume of coagulation factors, while the supplemented plasma (FFP) contains a larger volume. Supplementation of coagulation factors is necessary in patients with diseases such as liver failure or thrombotic microangiopathy.

1.2 Properties of Therapies Relating to Removal of Pathogenic Substances

1.2.1 Mechanisms of Elimination

The original modality of apheresis was exchange transfusion. In this procedure, blood containing pathogenic substances was drawn from the body and discarded, followed by infusion of the same quantity of pathogen-free donor blood.

With some apheresis modalities, only the pathogenic substance is removed, requiring a smaller quantity of blood product. These techniques employ diffusion, filtration, adsorp-

TABLE 1.2 Principles of removal employed in blood purification

	Advantages	**Disadvantages**
Diffusion (dialysis)	Larger clearance per session or per defined time	Limited clearance of larger molecules
	No reduction of blood volume	Requires dialysate
Filtration	Removal of larger molecules	Requires fluid supplementation
		Limited clearance compared with diffusion
Adsorption	No reduction of blood volume	Limited adsorption capacity
	Fluid supplementation and dialysate not required	Unclear mechanisms of substance adsorption
Centrifugation	Simplicity of devices	Requires fluid supplementation

tion or centrifugation to separate substances based on their physical or chemical properties. The removed blood is returned to the body and the patient receives blood product or albumin solution supplementation when necessary.

These earlier mentioned mechanisms are discussed in greater detail in the following sections; their properties, advantages, and shortcomings are summarized in Table 1.2.

1.2.1.1   Diffusion (Fig. 1.1a)

Elimination of solute through diffusion is the mechanism used in hemodialysis. Diffusion involves the passive movement of substances across a semipermeable membrane from a region of higher concentration to one of lower concentration. In hemodialysis, substances diffuse across the membrane based on differences in the concentrations of solutes in the plasma and dialysate. Therefore, the concentration of solute

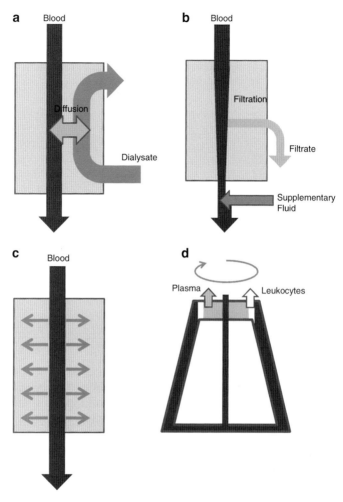

FIGURE 1.1 Properties of each principle. (**a**) Diffusion: substances move along the concentration gradient between plasma and dialysate; does not produce blood volume deficit and fluid supplementation is not required. (**b**) Filtration: target pathogenic substances are removed together with fluid; fluid supplementation is necessary to compensate for volume deficit. (**c**) Adsorption: target substances are adsorbed on blood purification devices; does not result in volume deficit or need for dialysate or fluid supplementation. (**d**) Centrifugation: plasma and cellular components are separated according to the differences in their specific gravity

within the dialysate is important for determining the efficacy of substance removal from the plasma.

Clearance by diffusion is determined by blood and dialysate flow rate and membrane properties. Increasing the dialysate flow rate as appropriate allows high clearance of substances from plasma; maximum clearance can theoretically be the same as plasma flow rate. Fluid deficit does not occur during dialysis, obviating the need for fluid supplementation. However, the efficacy of large molecule removal is low and large molecules such as albumin cannot be removed during dialysis treatment.

1.2.1.2   Filtration (Fig. 1.1b)

Large molecules that cannot be removed by hemodialysis (diffusion) can be removed through filtration. The two main types of filters are hemofilters and plasma separators. Albumin passes readily through plasma separators but poorly through hemofilters [1].

Hemofilters are used for molecules up to 20–30 kDa, while plasma separators are used in plasmapheresis to remove substances larger than albumin, which measures 67 kDa. Types of plasmapheresis include double filtration plasmapheresis (DFPP) and plasma adsorption (PA), in addition to simple plasma exchange. These modalities allow reduction in the blood product volume needed for fluid supplementation during plasmapheresis. Plasma fractionators are used in DFPP and plasma adsorptive columns are used for PA.

The efficacy of filtration is not as great as that of dialysis in terms of the per hour or per session removal of substances. We should eliminate the pathogenic molecules in forms where it is dissolved in fluid during filtration. Therefore, filtration always results in fluid volume reduction requiring fluid supplementation.

Most of the oncotic pressure in plasma is generated by albumin. Albumin removal by plasmapheresis requires FFP or albumin supplementation to maintain oncotic pressure. Hemofiltration also requires extracellular fluid replacement, although this technique does not remove a clinically significant amount of albumin.

Because both methods require an equivalent amount of fluid to that filtered, larger volume of supplementation is required if we intend to increase the clearance. Clearance of small solutes using filtration methods is limited primarily due to the high cost of blood products compared to the cost of hemodialysis.

The replacement fluid generally is infused after filtration. Filtration decreases the plasma volume at the filter outlet and concentrates the red blood cells. Therefore, the filtration fraction cannot be increased beyond half the plasma flow rate (usually 30 % of blood flow rate) [2]. In contrast, small solute clearance can theoretically be increased up to the plasma flow rate with hemodialysis. The clearance per time unit that can be attained by filtration cannot exceed that of hemodialysis.

Plasmapheresis generally is used to remove proteins such as autoantibodies, which have a small distribution volume. Plasmapheresis is sufficient to remove adequate amounts of these substances, even though clearance is limited.

1.2.1.3   Adsorption (Fig. 1.1c)

Adsorption is used to remove substances according to their physical properties, such as charge, hydrophobicity, or hydrophilicity. This method is in sharp contrast to filtration or dialysis in which molecular weight almost exclusively determines the efficacy of removal. Pores on the surface of the adsorptive material increase the material's surface area. The relationship between the pore size and molecular weight also determines the efficacy of removal.

Two types of devices are used for adsorption. In one type, the adsorption material itself is woven as a fabric or formed into beads. The second type consists of small molecule ligands that capture pathogenic substances that adhere to the resin carrier (Table 1.3). The devices also can be categorized according to the type of fluid to be perfused. A direct hemoperfusion column can be used with whole blood, while a plasma adsorptive column can only be used with separated plasma.

TABLE 1.3 Ligands and their specific target substances in adsorption

Principle of adsorption	Characteristics	Ligand	Carrier	Target substance	Product name
Physiochemical interaction	Electrostatic force	Dextran sulfate	Porous cellulose beads	Low density lipoprotein	Liposorber[a]
				Anti-cardiolipin antibody	Selesorb[a]
		Styrene divinylbenzene copolymer		Bilirubin, bile acid	Plasorba BRS[b]
	Hydrophobic adsorption	Tryptophan		Auto-antibodies	Immusorba TR[b]
		Phenylalanine		Immune complex	Immusorba PH[b]
		Activated charcoal		Toxins, drugs	Hemosorba[b]
		Hexadecyl group	Cellulose	β2 microglobulin	Lixelle[a]

(continued)

TABLE 1.3 (continued)

Principle of adsorption	Characteristics	Ligand	Carrier	Target substance	Product name
Biological interaction	Specific binding	Polymyxin B	α-Chloroacetoamide-methylated polystyrene fiber	Endotoxin	Toraymyxin[c]
				Cytokines	
	Adhesion molecules	Cellulose diacetate		Granulocytes, monocytes	Adacolumn[d]
		Polyester fibers		Leukocytes	Cellsorba[b]

Manufactures of each product:
[a]Kaneka Medix Co., Ltd., Osaka, Japan
[b]Asahi-kasei Medical Co., Ltd., Tokyo, Japan, Urayasu, Japan
[c]Toray Medical Co., Ltd
[d]Japan Immunoresearch Laboratories Co., Ltd., Takasaki, Japan

The adsorptive method has the advantage that fluid is not removed; thus, fluid supplementation is not necessary. Both types of columns have a maximum adsorption capacity. Once the amount of pathogenic substances exceeds this capacity, additional substance cannot be removed with the same column (Fig. 1.2). The adsorption capacity can be somewhat unpredictable depending on the substance to be removed; for example each subclass of IgG has a different adsorptive capacity in tryptophan conjugated column.

1.2.1.4   Centrifugation (Fig. 1.1d)

Centrifugation is used to separate cellular components from plasma. Cellular components, primarily red blood cells, form a sediment when anticoagulated blood is left still. The specific gravity of cellular components is greater than that of plasma. Removal of cellular components from plasma can be accomplished uniformly and in less time with the use of centrifugation methods.

Apheresis with centrifugation is used for removal of plasma (e.g., plasma exchange, popular in the United States), or separation of cellular components (e.g., leukocytapheresis, no longer reimbursed by the Japanese government), or cytapheresis for blood component transfusion, or for peripheral blood stem cell transplantation.

Plasma containing albumin is discarded together with the pathogenic substances during plasma exchange by centrifugation, as well as membrane separation. Fluid supplementation containing solutes that maintain oncotic pressure is necessary.

1.3   Properties of Removed Substances

1.3.1   Introduction

Properties of target substances are important for efficacy of removal and they determine selection of modality, dose of therapies, and frequency of therapies.

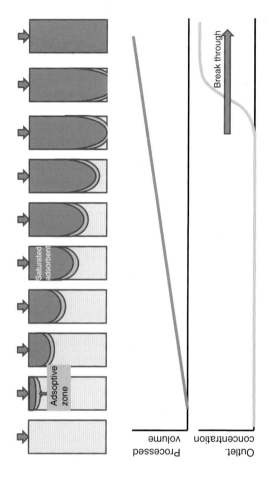

FIGURE 1.2 Process of adsorption. The adsorptive zone, where actual adsorption occurs, moves from the inlet to the outlet of the column. The adsorbent behind the adsorptive zone is fully occupied by target substances. Once the adsorptive zone reaches the outlet, target substances are detected in the fluid drained from the outlet (breakthrough)

TABLE 1.4 Substance characteristics and associated removal methods

Characteristics of substances	Diffusion	Filtration	Adsorption	Centrifugation
Distribution volume	O	O	O	O
Compartment	O	O	O	O
Half-life, production rate	O	O	O	O
Molecular weight	O	O	△	–
Charge	△	–	O	–
Hydrophilic or hydrophobic properties	△	–	O	–
Specific gravities	–	–	–	O

(O) Applicable, (△) partially applicable

These properties include both kinetic and physicochemical parameters (Table 1.4). Distribution volume, compartment, and half-life are important among kinetic parameters, while molecular weight, electric charge, hydrophilic or hydrophobic properties, and specific gravity are important among physicochemical properties. Kinetic parameters are described in Chapter 14, "Determination of therapeutic dose and frequency" on page. In this section, physicochemical factors are discussed from the perspective of modality selection.

1.3.2   Molecular Weight

The effects of molecular weight differ according to the selected modality. The relationship between device pore size and molecular weight affect removal efficacy by filtration and diffusion (dialysis).

The substances with molecular weight smaller than the cut-off weight limit for the device pass through the pores and are uniformly removed during filtration. Hemofiltration does not filter albumin, but substances with a molecular weight less than 20 kDa do cross the hemofilter. The membrane plasma separator does not filter cellular components within blood, but does allow LDL-cholesterol or substances of smaller size to pass through.

Substances are uniformly passed through the membrane irrespective of molecular weight as long as the molecular weight is less than the specific cut-off weight of each membrane. The second filters for double filtration plasmapheresis (DFPP) are available with different pore sizes. The pore size is selected based on the size needed to filter the specific pathogenic substance [3].

Diffusion removes substances to the degree that is negatively proportional to their molecular weight. Dialyzers usually do not pass albumin and have limited removal efficacy for larger molecules weighing 20 kDa or more, while smaller substances such as urea can easily be removed. However, even smaller substances cannot be removed by dialysis if they are attached to larger substances such as albumin [4].

Molecular weight differences also determine the specificity for substance removal using adsorption. For example, both Liposorber and Selesorb use the same ligand (dextran sulfate), but have different pore sizes. The difference in pore size determines the specificity of the two adsorptive columns; Selesorb adsorbs immune complexes and antibodies, while, Liposorber adsorbs the larger low-density lipoprotein molecule [5].

Figure 1.3 indicates the relationship between molecular weight and clearance per session under usual conditions for different modalities of blood purification therapy. The figure illustrates either the modality or the effect of molecular weight on the clearance per session. Molecules larger than albumin can only be removed by plasmapheresis even though the clearance is low. Therefore, small solutes such as urea certainly can be removed through plasmapheresis, but

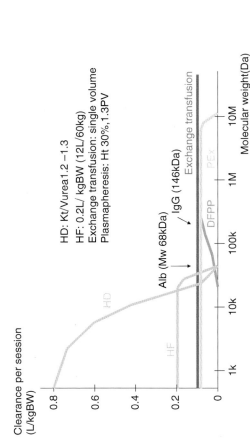

FIGURE 1.3 The relationship between molecular weight and clearance per session with various modalities for ordinary therapeutic uses. Clearance of each modality per session differs according to molecular weight. The clearance of hemodialysis is highest for smaller substances, while substances larger than albumin can be removed solely by plasmapheresis, although clearance is limited. HD: hemodialysis, HF: hemofiltration, BW: body weight, PV: plasma volume, Ht: hematocrit, Alb: albumin, DFPP: double filtration plasma pheresis, PEx: simple plasma exchange

efficiency is quite low because of its low clearance and the requirement for blood derived products. In contrast, IgG (Mw: 150 kDa) cannot be removed by hemodialysis or hemofiltration, because it does not pass through the dialyzer due to its size.

1.3.3   Properties That Affect Adsorption

Electric charge: Some molecules have an electric charge. Molecules with opposite charges attract each other, while those with the same charge repulse each other. Therefore, substances within plasma with a positive charge are absorbed by a negatively charged ligand.

Hydrophobicity or hydrophilicity: Water molecules are electrically charged. Therefore, substances that have a charge or polarity are attracted by water and are considered hydrophilic. Substances without a charge or polarity are not attracted by water and are considered hydrophobic (Fig. 1.4).

Hydrophobicity or hydrophilicity are important properties affecting adsorptive procedures. Hydrophobic substances rarely exist within a water solution alone, but are attracted to hydrophobic ligands on adsorptive columns and removed from the plasma as it passes through the column.

1.3.4   Specific Gravity and Centrifugation

The specific gravity of plasma is between 1.025 and 1.029, which is smaller than the specific gravities of blood cells (Table 1.5). Therefore, anticoagulant-treated blood separates into the plasma component above the blood cell component when the blood is left still. With centrifugation, separation occurs more rapidly and uniformly. Centrifugation gates that separate blood cells and plasma or a buffy coat containing white cells and platelets from other components are generally used for plasma separation and cytapheresis.

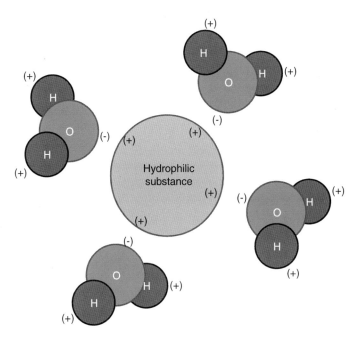

FIGURE 1.4 Hydrophilic substances in water. Water molecules have polarity. Charged substances are attracted to water molecules. Such substances are called hydrophilic

TABLE 1.5 Specific gravities of plasma and cellular blood components

Substances or cellular components	Specific gravity
Plasma	1.025–1.029
Platelets	1.04
White blood cells	1.050–1.092
Red blood cells	1.078–1.114

Note: Removal by Biologically Specific Reactions
Antigen-antibody reactions are used to remove pathogenic antibodies. A column with immobilized A or B blood type antigens can be used to remove anti-A or anti-B antibodies, respectively. Peptides of acetylcholine receptors (AchR) are immobilized by a column that captures anti-AchR antibodies. Such biologic reactions are highly specific. Pathogenic substances can be removed without affecting other substances when using highly specific reactions. Higher cost, safety concerns, and storage stability preclude the clinical use of this technique in Japan.

References

1. Hirata N et al (2003) Plasma separator plasmaflo OP. Ther Apher Dial 7(1):64–68
2. Gurland HJ et al (1984) Comparative evaluation of filters used in membrane plasmapheresis. Nephron 36(3):173–182
3. Nakaji S et al (2002) Membranes for therapeutic apheresis. Ther Apher 6(4):267–270
4. Maher JF (1977) Principles of dialysis and dialysis of drugs. Am J Med 62(4):475–481
5. Hidaka T et al (1999) Evaluation of adsorption selectivity dextran sulfate bound cellulose beads for the removal of anti-DNA antibodies. Ther Apher 3(1):75–80

Chapter 2
Methods to Remove Pathogens

Tamami Tanaka, Osamu Ichimura, Yugo Nagae, and Nobuhiro Sakuma

Main Points

Membrane

- Membrane fractionation is the main technique used to separate pathogens in apheresis therapy.
- Molecules are separated by the pore size of the membrane's surface.
- Because pathogens and water are removed, substitution fluid is generally necessary.

T. Tanaka (✉)
Department of Hemodialysis and Apheresis, University Hospital,
The University of Tokyo, 7-3-1 Hongo, Bunkyo-ku, Tokyo 113-8655, Japan

Kitasenju Higashiguchi Kidney Clinic, 1F Gakuen-dori Bldg. 11-2,
Senjuasahicho, Adachi-ku, Tokyo 120-0026, Japan
e-mail: tfukue-tky@umin.ac.jp

N. Sakuma • O. Ichimura • Y. Nagae
Department of Medical Engineering, University Hospital,
The University of Tokyo, 7-3-1 Hongo, Bunkyo-ku, Tokyo 113-8655, Japan

E. Noiri and N. Hanafusa (eds.), *The Concise Manual*
of Apheresis Therapy, DOI 10.1007/978-4-431-54412-8_2,
© Springer Japan 2014

21

Adsorption
- Adsorption is a physical property used in direct hemoperfusion and plasma adsorption.
- Adsorption can be divided into selective adsorption and nonselective adsorption. Selective adsorption exploits specific physiochemical properties that may differ with each substance such as hydrophobic and electrostatic interactions. Nonselective absorption uses activated carbon.
- Adsorbents are porous to increase the surface area for adsorption and to separate the substances by the pore size.

Centrifugation
- Centrifugation is a separation method that uses the different specific gravities of plasma and blood cells to differentiate them.
- There are two kinds of centrifugation methods: intermittent flow and continuous flow.
- Centrifugation is commonly used for peripheral blood stem cell harvesting and processing donated blood. While this technique can be used for plasma exchange, that is rarely done.

2.1   Membrane

2.1.1   Introduction

The membrane fractionation technique for hemodialysis has been applied to the treatment of various diseases, such as autoimmune diseases, and has led to the development of a therapeutic system of apheresis.

The main techniques utilized are plasma separation (the separation of blood cells from plasma) and plasma component fractionation (the selective removal of pathogens). This chapter presents the basics of membrane fractionation.

2.1.2   Characteristics of Membrane Fractionation

All of the plasma separators, plasma component fractionators, and hemofilters used in hemofiltration separate the substances in the solution by generating hydrostatic pressure that drives substances toward the pores. The size, represented by the molecular weight, of the substance regulates whether it is filtered or not. Because substances will be removed along with water molecules, fluid replacement is necessary. For example, crystalloid solution is replaced in hemofiltration, and albumin is replaced in plasma separation and plasma component fractionation, to maintain physiologic colloid osmotic pressure (Fig. 2.1).

2.1.2.1   Pore Size

The molecular weight of a substance determines whether it will be able to pass through the size of the pores on the filter membrane. Substances smaller than the pore size can pass through the filter, but bigger substances cannot.

2.1.2.2   Sieving Coefficient

The sieving coefficient (SC) is an important term in membrane fractionation. SC is the ratio of the concentration in the filtrate (CF) to the concentration in the blood inlets (CBi). For example, the SC of a substance that is small enough to pass through the filter is 1. The SC of a substance that is bigger than the pore size and cannot be filtered at all is 0.

$$SC = \frac{CF}{CBi}$$

2.1.3   Example of Membrane Fractionation

2.1.3.1   Plasma Separation

Plasma separation can be accomplished by using membrane fractionation or centrifugal separation. Nowadays membrane

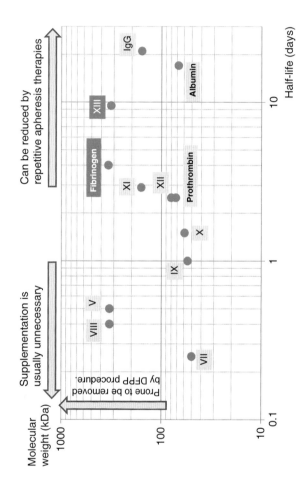

FIGURE 2.1 Diagram showing the relationship between molecular weight and half-life of the substances in apheresis therapy

fractionation is the main plasma separation technique used for therapy in Japan because of the small blood filler content, efficiency, low cost, ease of handling the equipment, and other considerations.

Separating molecules by membrane fractionation allows plasma components smaller than the pores (pore diameter of about 0.3 mm) [1] to pass, but will not pass bigger components such as red or white blood cells, lymphocytes, or platelets. The SC of albumin and globulin in plasma is 1 in theory, so substances with a molecular weight of less than about 150–200×10^4 Da [2] can be separated (Fig. 2.2).

Plasma exchange (PE) is a plasma separation procedure that removes the separated plasma, including pathogens, and exchanges it with a replacement fluid (Fig. 2.3a). Another type of plasma separation procedure filters the separated plasma through an adsorbent, for cases where direct hemoperfusion is inadequate (Fig. 2.3b).

2.1.3.2   Plasma Component Fractionation

A plasma component fractionator can further separate plasma produced from plasma separation. Large molecules such as immunoglobulins and LDL-cholesterol can be separated selectively, concentrated, and discarded, and smaller molecules like albumin can be returned to a patient's body efficiently.

This procedure of separating plasma from the blood, and then further separating the plasma through plasma component fractionation, is called DFPP (double filtration plasmapheresis), because both plasma separation and plasma component fractionation are utilized (Fig. 2.4).

The practical separation of albumin, globulin, and pathogens by a plasma fractionator is not completely satisfactory. This is because the molecular sizes are similar (Fig. 2.2) and the membrane pore size is uneven to some extent. Variations of this procedure, such as cryofiltration, have been developed to reduce this inefficiency.

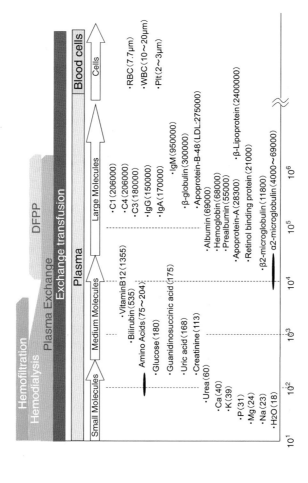

FIGURE 2.2 Molecular weight of endogenous substances encountered in various apheresis therapies [3]

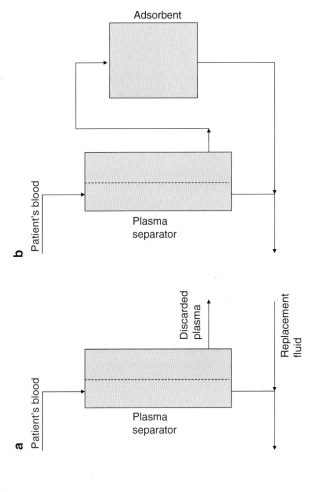

FIGURE 2.3 Diagram of plasma exchange (**a**) and plasma adsorption (**b**)

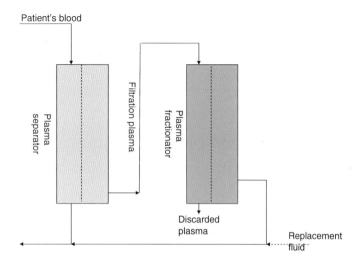

FIGURE 2.4 Double filtration plasmapheresis

2.1.4   Separators

All membrane plasma separators and plasma component fractionators on the market (Table 2.1) have hollow fiber membranes and resemble dialyzers that are used for hemodialysis, but these techniques differ from each other in their membrane pore sizes. The pore size of a membrane plasma separator differs by 0.1 mm, and that of a plasma component fractionator used to separate albumin and globulin differs by 0.01 mm.

2.2   Adsorption

2.2.1   Introduction

Hemodialysis and apheresis therapy is based on various physical phenomenon such as diffusion, filtration, adsorption, and others. This chapter presents therapy based on adsorption.

TABLE 2.1 The list of plasma separators and plasma fractionators

Company	Product name	Model	Hollow fiber material	Effective surface (m²)	Pore size (mm)	Inside diameter (mm)	Wall thickness (mm)	Priming volume (mL)	Maximum pressure (mm Hg)
Plasma separator									
Asahi Kasei Medical	Plasmaflo	OP-02W	Polyethylene	0.2	0.30	350	50	25	60
		OP-05W		0.5	0.30	350	50	55	60
		OP-08W		0.8	0.30	350	50	80	60
Kawasumi Laboratories	Plasmacure	PE-02	Polyethylene	0.2	0.30	330	50	25	60
		PE-05		0.5	0.30	330	50	55	60
		PE-08		0.8	0.30	330	50	80	60
	Evacure	1A10	Ethylene vinyl alcohol copolymer	1.0	0.008	175	40	125	250
		2A10		1.0	0.01	175	40	125	250
		3A10		1.0	0.02	175	40	125	250
		4A10		1.0	0.03	175	40	125	250
		1A20		2.0	0.008	175	40	125	250
		2A20		2.0	0.01	175	40	125	250
		3A20		2.0	0.02	175	40	125	250
		4A20		2.0	0.03	175	40	125	250

(continued)

TABLE 2.1 (continued)

Company	Product name	Model	Hollow fiber material	Effective surface (m²)	Pore size (mm)	Inside diameter (mm)	Wall thickness (mm)	Priming volume (mL)	Maximum pressure (mm Hg)
Kaneka Medix Corp.	Sulflux	FP-02	Polyethylene	0.2	0.30	350	50	25	60
		FP-05		0.5	0.30	350	50	55	60
		FP-08		0.8	0.30	350	50	80	60
Plasma fractionator									
Asahi Kasei Medical	Cascadeflo	EC-20W	Ethylene vinyl alcohol	2.0	0.01	220	80	130	500
		EC-30W		2.0	0.02	220	80	130	500
		EC-40W		2.0	0.03	220	80	130	500
		EC-50W		2.0	0.03	220	80	130	500
Kawasumi Laboratories	Evaflux	2A10	Ethylene vinyl alcohol copolymer	1.0	0.01	175	40	100	500
		4A10		1.0	0.03	175	40	100	500
		2A20		2.0	0.01	175	40	140	500
		3A20		2.0	0.02	175	40	140	500
		4A20		2.0	0.03	175	40	140	500
		5A20		2.0	0.03	175	40	140	500

The purpose of adsorption is to decrease a pathogen's concentration in the blood to improve a patient's condition. Adsorption using ion exchange resin was performed for a patient suffering hepatic encephalopathy by Scechter in 1958 for the first time, and its indications as a therapy have expanded to various other diseases thanks to the development of various adsorbents.

2.2.2   Categorization by the Difference of Perfusion

Adsorption is used in direct hemoperfusion and plasma adsorption. Both procedures can remove only pathogens and do not affect blood or plasma volume. Therefore fluid or cell supplementation is not necessary.

2.2.2.1   Direct Hemoperfusion

This technique involves passing large volumes of blood directly over the adsorbent. This method is simple, because specific equipment beyond an apparatus for hemodialysis is not required. However, direct contact between the adsorbent and the blood cells may cause the capture and degeneration of blood components. Furthermore, the columns tend to cause coagulation due to platelet activation.

2.2.2.2   Plasma Adsorption

In this technique, plasma and pathogens are separated from whole blood cells first before the adsorption process. A dedicated device is necessary and the apparatus is complicated. However, direct contact between blood cells and the adsorbent is avoided. Additionally, adsorbents with slightly less biocompatibility may be used.

2.2.3   How to Adsorb

There are two kinds of adsorption: selective adsorption by ligands and nonselective adsorption. Ligands selectively bind to specific proteins or receptors on a cell membrane. Selective adsorption requires the ligands to bind only to the target pathogens by means of a physiochemical biological interaction. Alternatively, nonselective adsorption uses the adsorptive material's natural attractive power, such as that which activated carbon possesses. Thus, the removal efficiency of the adsorption process depends not on the pathogen's molecular weight, but on the chemical nature of the pathogens, which differs from separation techniques used in diffusion and filtration.

Adsorbents have an upper limit on the amount of substance they can adsorb. Therefore, the surface of an adsorbent is porous to increase the exposure to the ligands and to separate adsorbed pathogens, which improves the efficiency of pathogen removal.

2.2.4   The Characteristics of Adsorbents

2.2.4.1   Adsorbents with Ligands

Physiochemical interactions have two important actions, hydrophobic bonding and electrostatic bonding. Hydrophobic bonding action is the action based on van der Waals force that describes how hydrophobic substances in a solution approach each other to avoid contact with water. The electrostatic bonding action is described by Coulomb's law that explains how negative and positive charges behave when approaching each other.

The biological interaction has two major components. One is the action based on antigen-antibody reactions, and the other is the action based on biological bonding reactions between receptors and ligands. Nowadays these types of adsorbent columns are not for sale in Japan.

Biological adsorbents are superior to physiochemical adsorbents in selectivity and specificity for pathogens. However, biological adsorbents can be difficult to sterilize and maintain, and can cause allergic reactions to the ligands. To minimize these problems, some adsorbents have biological structures that are compounds of chemical peptides.

Although physiochemical adsorbents are inferior to biological adsorbents in selectivity and specificity, a greater range of pathogens can be removed. The selectivity and specificity can be improved by optimizing the adsorbent's porosity and pore size.

2.2.4.2   Nonselective Adsorbents

Activated carbon is a form of nonselective adsorbent that will not adsorb specific pathogens nor support ligand interactions. Active carbon derived from petroleum pitch is now common, and these carbons are coated with a biocompatible material, such as poly-HEMA (poly-hydroxyethyl-methacrylate). These type of adsorbents, which adsorb 100–5,000 Da molecules, have not been used as a first choice recently because of the introduction of high performance membranes, and they are mainly used for patients suffering from addiction. (See Chap. 36)

2.3   Centrifugation

2.3.1   Introduction

Centrifugation is a separation method using centrifugal force and specific gravity.

Whole blood cells and anticoagulants are added to the centrifugal bowl, which looks like a hanging bell. Centrifugal force is produced by high-speed rotation (maximum 6,000 rpm).

Centrifugal force drives substances away from the center of rotation, and substances are acted upon according to their

TABLE 2.2 Specific gravity of blood components

Substance	Specific gravity	Position in centrifugation bowl
Plasma	1.025–1.029	Move to center
Platelet	1.040	
WBC	1.050–1.092	
RBC	1.078–1.114	Move to edge

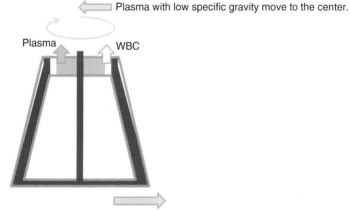

Plasma with low specific gravity move to the center.

Plasma   WBC

Substance with high specific gravity move to the edge.

FIGURE 2.5 Whole blood components are separated in a gradient from the center to the edge in centrifugation bowl according to their specific gravity. Thus, selected blood components can be removed

specific gravity, with heavier material moving farther toward the edge. Table 2.2 shows the specific gravity of blood components. Target pathogens can also be separated by using this method (Fig. 2.5).

2.3.2   Characteristics

2.3.2.1   Comparison with Membrane Separation Method

Centrifugation has certain advantages:

- Substances' separability is good.
- Only target pathogens can be collected and removed.
- Peripheral veins can be used as vascular access.
- Separation membranes are not necessary.

    There are also disadvantages:

- Platelets cannot be separated completely from the plasma.
- Specific equipment is necessary, which differs from the requirements for common membrane separation.

2.3.2.2   Difference Between Intermittent and Continuous Flow Centrifugation

Centrifugation may use intermittent or continuous flow techniques, so named for the way the blood is withdrawn and returned.

The intermittent flow method requires only one venipuncture site, because the same line is used to both collect and return the blood. This method needs more time and a larger priming volume, so it is not suitable for light weight patients such as children.

Continuous flow centrifugation requires two venipuncture sites to collect and return blood simultaneously. A large blood volume can be treated at one time in spite of a small priming volume. This method is not suitable for patients who have difficulty with venipuncture. This treatment also requires the restriction of patient movements, which can be stressful for some patients.

2.3.2.3   Points to Note

Centrifugation often requires sodium citrate (ACD-A fluid) as an anticoagulant. ACD-A fluid is typically mixed with the whole blood cells in a ratio of 1 to 10–13. A large volume of sodium citrate can cause both hypocalcemia and an increase in extracellular fluid volume, so calcium replacement is often necessary (see Chap. 16).

2.3.3   Target Indications for Centrifugation

The centrifugation method is commonly used for separation of donated blood products.

2.3.3.1   Separation of Blood Cells

Peripheral blood stem cells, platelets, and white blood cells (WBCs) can be separated through centrifugation. It can be used to collect peripheral blood stem cells for peripheral blood stem cell transplantation, because the damage or activation of blood cells is rare. This method can also be used for the collection of platelets for platelet donation. (See Chap. 38)

2.3.3.2   Separation of Plasma

Centrifugation is performed to separate plasma for plasma donation (FFP) and treatment. In the plasma exchange process, plasma separated by centrifugation is discarded, and the same volume of albumin or FFP are supplied. However, membrane fractionation is common in Japan, so plasma exchange is mostly performed by this method and not by centrifugation.

Note: Buffy Coat

The buffy coat is the white layer of WBCs and platelets between the layer of plasma and that of red blood cells that forms after density gradient centrifugation. This layer includes layers of platelets, lymphocytes, monocytes, and granulocytes in order of increasing density gradient, allowing target substances to be collected and removed.

References

1. Hirata N et al (2003) Ther Apher Dial 7:64–68
2. Iwamoto H (2009) Jin to Toseki, vol 65, p 212
3. Kaneko I (2004) Ketuekijokaryoho handbook, Kyodo Isho Shuppan,Tokyo, pp 6–7

Chapter 3
Decision to Prescribe PE, DFPP, or PA

Rei Isshiki and Hiroko Yamamoto

> **Main Points**
> - Plasmapheresis modalities include: plasma exchange (PE), double filtration plasmapheresis (DFPP), and plasma adsorption (PA).
> - A goal of apheresis is to minimize the amount of blood-derived products used for therapy.
> - PA removes targeted substances with the highest level of specificity, followed in descending order by DFPP and PE.

3.1   Introduction

Plasmapheresis modalities include plasma exchange (PE), double filtration plasmapheresis (DFPP), and plasma adsorption (PA). Apheresis has been developed to decrease the

R. Isshiki (✉) • H. Yamamoto
Department of Hemodialysis and Apheresis, University Hospital,
University of Tokyo, 7-3-1 Hongo, Bunkyo-ku, Tokyo 113-8655, Japan
e-mail: risshiki-tky@umin.ac.jp

E. Noiri and N. Hanafusa (eds.), *The Concise Manual
of Apheresis Therapy,* DOI 10.1007/978-4-431-54412-8_3,
© Springer Japan 2014

volume of blood-derived products used in therapy; the three major modalities differ in this respect. This chapter presents the advantages and disadvantages of each modality and the current knowledge with respect to prescribing optimum therapeutic apheresis.

3.2   Plasmapheresis Modalities

3.2.1   Plasma Exchange

PE involves the removal of separated plasma and subsequent supplementation with the same amount of plasma fraction or fresh frozen plasma (FFP). Complete plasma exchange allows removal of a wider range of pathogenic substances than the other two modalities. Additionally, coagulation factors and normal immunoglobulin can be recovered when FFP is used for fluid supplementation.

Disadvantages of PE include the requirement for fluid supplementation equal to the volume of discarded plasma and a higher risk of transfusion-transmitted diseases and allergies than is seen with the other therapies. Because a large volume of sodium citrate preservative is injected with FFP, hemodialysis combination therapy should be considered to remove sodium, correct the acid–base balance, and replenish calcium [1].

PE should be considered for first-line therapy in:

Patients with hepatic failure, to replenish coagulation factors

Patients with thrombotic thrombocytopenic purpura (TTP) or hemolytic uremic syndrome (HUS), to replenish disintegrin and metalloproteinase with thrombospondin type 1 motifs 13 (ADAMTS-13) [2]

Patients who have active bleeding, such as alveolar hemorrhage, or infection, to prevent active bleeding or infection due to the reduction of coagulation factors and normal immunoglobulin that occurs with DFPP and PA [3]

3.2.2   Other Therapies

When performing plasmapheresis using the DFPP or PA method, the Practitioner should estimate the quantity of pathogenic substance in plasma before selecting the plasma separator (DFPP) or adsorption column (PA). Fluid supplementation is not required with some types of plasmapheresis.

3.2.2.1   Double Filtration Plasmapheresis

The purpose of the second plasma filtration step of DFPP is to separate useful substances (primarily albumin) from high molecular weight pathogenic substances. The filtered albumin-rich solution is then reintroduced into the blood stream via the venous port.

DFPP is designed to selectively remove immunoglobulins (IgG, IgA, IgM, IgD, and IgE) from the plasma. The immunoglobulins differ in molecular weight (IgM [970,000] > [IgE > IgD >]   IgA   [160,000] > IgG   [140,000–170,000]) and in blood concentration (IgG [70–75 %] > IgA [10–15 %] > IgM [10 %] > IgE and IgD [<1 %]) IgG is the most commonly targeted immunoglobulin.

An advantage of DFPP is the capability to separate useful substances from pathogenic ones based on differences in molecular weight, with subsequent removal of the pathogenic substances and return of the useful substances to the bloodstream. DFPP requires less fluid supplementation compared to that of PE (e.g., one-fifth of the fluid volume and one-third of the albumin are needed with EC-20W) because only some of the processed plasma is discarded. Each of the four types of second filters (plasma fractionators) available in Japan requires a different volume of supplementary fluid depending on the filter pore size.

A disadvantage of DFPP is that the performance of its second filter is not high enough to remove all of the IgG (particularly small molecular weight IgG), while some albumin is removed and discarded. Additionally, substances smaller than albumin cannot be removed by DFPP and are returned to the blood; however, these substances may be removed by hemofiltration.

Even though the volume of waste fluid is small, it contains large amounts of high oncotic pressure substances; therefore FFP cannot be used for fluid supplementation because of its lower oncotic pressure. Concentrated albumin is used for fluid supplementation in most cases [4].

Additionally, coagulation factors and normal immunoglobulins cannot be replenished with DFPP because of the use of albumin for fluid supplementation, resulting in reduction of these substances with therapy. Fluid supplementation often is not needed with removal of high-molecular-weight substances such as LDL or hepatitis C virus using the DFPP method.

DFPP should be considered for first-line therapy in the following circumstances:

Patients with autoimmune disease, because they do not need coagulation factor or normal immunoglobulin replenishment.
Patients awaiting renal homotransplantation and those with a blood type incompatible pregnancy, because blood product use should be avoided in these patients, who are often young.
Patients with multiple myeloma or macroglobulinemia for treatment of hyperviscosity syndrome (with increasing IgM levels).
Patients with a high LDL-cholesterol level, in whom efficiency increases with use of the double-filtration plasmapheresis thermo-mode.
Patients with chronic hepatitis C, for virus removal and eradication (VRAD) when combined with interferon therapy (for details, refer to "4.5 HCV infection") [5].

3.2.2.2   Plasma Adsorption

PA involves plasma separation by the first membrane (plasma separator) followed by plasma delivery to the adsorption column, where pathogenic substances are adsorbed via hydrophobic or electrostatic adsorption interactions.

Fluid supplementation is not required with PA because the plasma volume remains the same and albumin is not adsorbed; thus, the oncotic pressure does not change. Four types of adsorption column ligands are available in Japan.

A disadvantage of PA is that its adsorption capability largely depends on the physical properties of the pathogenic substance to be removed. While all subtypes of IgG can be removed with DFPP, only certain IgG subtypes are removed with PA. For example, IgG_3 is especially well adsorbed by PA with a tryptophan-conjugated column but IgG_4 is not well adsorbed [3].

Additionally, the PA column generally can process a maximum volume of only 2–3 L of plasma (excepting some columns such as LA-15, which can be reactivated and used again). Therefore, PA is not suitable for patients with a large physique because of the larger volume of plasma to be processed [3].

PA should be considered for first-line therapy in the following circumstances:

Patients who cannot or hesitate to receive any blood-derived products.

Patients with a high LDL-cholesterol level, because of the high adsorption capability of the column and the large plasma volume that can be processed with the LA-15 column.

Targeted substances are removed with the highest level of specificity by PA, followed in descending order by DFPP and PE. If the therapy is not effective with one method, use of a different modality should be considered.

The characteristics of each plasmapheresis modality are summarized in Table 3.1.

Indications for therapeutic apheresis in Japan are shown in Table 3.2.

TABLE 3.1 The characteristics of each modality

	Advantage	Disadvantage	Usage of blood-derived products	Targeted substances
PE	Removes more types of pathogenic substances Replenishes normal plasma	High risk of transfusion transmitted disease	Large volume	Wide range
DFPP	Preserves albumin	Loss of coagulation factors and normal immunoglobulin	Small to medium volume	Substances larger than albumin
PA	Fluid supplementation not required	Processes limited plasma volume	Not required	Specific substances

TABLE 3.2 Indications for therapeutic apheresis in Japan

| | Plasma separator | Plasma fractionator | |
| | | Membrane | Adsorption |
	PE	DFPP	PA
1	Multiple myeloma	○	○	
2	Macroglobulinemia	○	○	
3	Fulminant hepatitis	○		limited[a]
4	Drug overdose	○		
5	Myasthenia gravis	○	○	○
6	Malignant rheumatoid arthritis	○	○	○
7	Systemic lupus erythematosus	○	○	○
8	Thrombotic thrombocytopenic purpura	○		
9	Blood type incompatible pregnancy	○	○	
10	Postoperative liver failure	○		limited[a]
11	Acute liver failure	○		limited[a]
12	Multiple sclerosis	○	○	○
13	Chronic inflammatory demyelinating polyneuropathy	○	○	○

(continued)

TABLE 3.2 (continued)

| | Plasma separator | Plasma fractionator | | Adsorption |
| | | Membrane | | |
	PE	DFPP		PA
14 Guillain–Barre syndrome	○	○		○
15 Pemphigus/pemphigoid	○	○		
16 Focal segmental glomerulosclerosis	○	○		○
17 Hemolytic uremic syndrome	○			
18 Familial hypercholesterolemia	○	○		○
19 Peripheral arterial disease	○	○		○
20 Renal homotransplantation	○	○		

[a]Bilirubin adsorption therapy may be performed in some cases, but only rarely because coagulation factors cannot be replenished and toxic substances metabolized by the liver cannot be removed

References

1. Abe T, Kobata H, Hanba Y et al (2004). Study of plasma exchange for liver failure: beneficial and harmful effects. Ther Apher Dial 8:180–4
2. Gail A. Rock, Kenneth H. Shumak, Noel A. Buskard et al (1991). Comparison of plasma exchange with plasma infusion in the treatment of thrombotic thrombocytopenic purpura. N Engl J Med 325:393–397
3. Hanafusa N (2011). Theoretical basis of pathogenic substance removal during plasmapheresis. Ther Apher Dial 15(5):421–430
4. Mineshima M, Agishi T, Hasuo Y et al (1992). Optimum albumin concentration of supplementation fluid for double filtration plasmapheresis. Artif Organs 16(5):510–3
5. Fujiwara K, Kaneko S, Kakumu S et al (2007). Double filtration plasmapheresis and interferon combination therapy for chronic hepatitis C patients with genotype 1 and high viral load. Hepatol Res 37: 701–10

Chapter 4
Plasma Exchange

Daisuke Katagiri and Hideo Kurosawa

> **Main Points**
> - Plasma exchange (PE) involves the withdrawal of blood from the circulation, centrifugal separation of the blood into plasma and cells, and return of the cellular components suspended in an inert medium.
> - Fresh frozen plasma (FFP) is used for replacement of proteins (with the exception of albumin), such as clotting factors.
> - The combination of PE and hemodialysis (HD) may be used to avoid development of hypocalcemia or hyponatremia caused by FFP.

D. Katagiri (✉)
Department of Nephrology & Endocrinology,
University Hospital, The University of Tokyo, 7-3-1 Hongo,
Bunkyo-ku, Tokyo 113-8655, Japan
e-mail: dkatagiri-tky@umin.ac.jp

H. Kurosawa
Department of Hemodialysis & Apheresis,
University Hospital, The University of Tokyo, 7-3-1 Hongo,
Bunkyo-ku, Tokyo 113-8655, Japan

E. Noiri and N. Hanafusa (eds.), *The Concise Manual
of Apheresis Therapy,* DOI 10.1007/978-4-431-54412-8_4,
© Springer Japan 2014

4.1   Introduction

PE involves the removal of blood from the circulation, followed by separation of blood cells and other substances from the plasma by centrifugation (based on cell density) or ultrafiltration using large-pore hemofilters (based on molecular size). This method is used to remove pathogenic substances, including autoreactive antibodies, immune complexes, paraproteins, lipoproteins, and inflammatory mediators such as cytokines. Fluid replacement after PE maintains normal plasma volume and electrolyte concentrations.

Do electrolytes get depleted through plasma removal?

4.2   Circuit and Preparation

Two methods are used to separate substances from plasma: centrifugation and membrane separation. For details, please refer to Table 2.1. Plasma filters have a pore size of about 0.3 mm and membrane area of 0.1–0.8 m². Homogenization of pore size has been sought to reduce cell leakage and hemolysis The plasmapheresis circuit includes the plasma filter, blood cell side circuit, plasma side circuit, equipment for plasma exchange [blood pump, plasma pump, hemadynamometer, plasma filtration manometer, and trans-membrane-pressure (TMP) manometer], and anticoagulant pump. A circuit for fluid replacement should be prepared when HD or hemodiafiltration is combined with PE. One of the following solutions should be prepared for PE: (a) 1,000 mL of normal saline and 1,000 mL of normal saline plus 1,000 U of heparin, or (b) 1,000 mL of normal saline and 1,000 mL of normal saline plus 40 mg of nafamostat mesilate.

4.3   Choice of Replacement Solution

The ideal replacement solution should maintain normovolemia and normal plasma electrolyte concentrations. The choice of replacement fluid includes crystalloids, semisynthetic colloids (hetastarch, gelatin, and dextrans), human albumin solutions, liquid stored plasma, fresh-frozen plasma (FFP), and cryoprecipitate. The replacement solutions most commonly used are liquid stored plasma and human albumin solution for removal of some pathogenic substances. FFP is often used for patients who need blood coagulation factor replenishment, such as those with hepatic failure, or for patients with thrombotic microangiopathy who need replacement of von Willebrand factor cleaving protease (vWFCP).

4.4   Adverse Effects of FFP Replenishment

FFP infusion can cause hypocalcemia as a result of calcium chelation by sodium citrate. Alkalosis and sodium overload can also occur. The hypotensive effects of citrate-induced hypocalcemia can be minimized by administering a calcium gluconate continuous intravenous infusion and monitoring serum calcium levels. The treatment of choice for patients with acute kidney injury (AKI) is combined plasmapheresis and HD to correct electrolyte abnormalities and provide renal support (see NOTE at end of chapter).

4.5   Clinical Application of PE

The typical PE procedure is performed at a 60–120 mL/min blood flow rate. The maximum rate for plasma separation is 30 % of the blood flow rate. Faster separation can lead to an increased risk of hypocalcemia, while slower separation can cause coagulation within the circuit. The blood flow rate should be restricted when using a superficial vein for vascular access. In general, the plasma separation rate and replenishment rate are equal.

4.6   Anticoagulant

Heparin is commonly used for anticoagulation in patients without a known bleeding disorder. The dose is 1,500 U for the first dose and 1,500–2,000 U/h for continuous dosing.

Anticoagulation is monitored by activated clotting time (ACT), with a target range of 150–180 s. Nafamostat mesilate administered at 20–50 mg/h is used in patients with bleeding disorders.

citrate Dosing

4.7 Complications of PE

Complications in addition to hypocalcemia and sodium overload include hypotension, bleeding, and allergic reaction with FFP replacement. *N/a overload. 2*
d/T Saline infusion?

4.7.1 Hypotension

The difference between the colloid oncotic pressure of the replacement fluid and that of the patient's plasma can cause hypotension. Monitoring changes in the colloid oncotic pressure using Crit-Line In-Line Monitor™ [In-Line Diagnostics, Kaysville, UT] is recommended. In patients with increased intravascular volume, albumin or replacement solution with a higher protein concentration should be considered to decrease the difference of oncotic pressure. In patients with low intravascular volume, replacement solution with a lower protein concentration should be considered.

4.7.2 Bleeding

Replacement with albumin may exacerbate bleeding because albumin solutions lack clotting factor. For details, please refer to Chap. 18.

4.7.3 Allergic Reaction

Patients may have an allergic reaction to nafamostat mesilate or FFP. For details, please refer to Chap. 19.

4.8   Points to Note

4.8.1   Immediately After Initiation of Therapy

Monitor the procedure to detect and prevent leakage of separated plasma caused by breach of the plasma filter. Ensure that fluid replacement is not interrupted by obstruction of the circuit.

4.8.2   During Therapy

A problem with the vascular access, drip chamber, or plasma filter should be considered if a patient develops elevated arterial or venous pressure. The use of an indwelling catheter for vascular access can result in the following problems: (a) circuit narrowing or obstruction with blood clotting, or (b) elevated interior pressure of the circuit and poor blood removal due to adhesion of the catheter to the blood vessel wall.

Clotting at the filter pores or at the plasma side of the filter should be suspected if an abrupt increase in TMP (transmembrane pressure) occurs. Adjusting the anticoagulant dose or infusing normal saline while monitoring TMP should alleviate the problem. The liquid level at the plasma side of the filter should be lowered. Changing the plasma filter should also be considered.

It is important to avoid hemolysis during plasma separation. Hemolysis with change of TMP has a greatly reduced number. The rate of plasma separation should be less than 30 % of the blood flow rate; TMP should be kept below 50 mmHg. The faster blood flow will lead lesser hemolysis with concentration of cell to the central of hollow fiber.

Can a newly inserted cvc bleed around insertion site = AC

How common is hemolysis?
How is it recognized?
what are interventions?

Note: Combination of PE with HD and Hemo-diafiltration

HD and plasma filtration should be combined using a serial connection to provide renal support or remove sodium citrate for the prevention of hypocalcemia and sodium overload in patients with renal dysfunction (Fig. 4.1). The priming volume is about 300 mL.

A high flow volume may be needed when combining hemodialysis or hemodiafiltration with PE in patients undergoing long-term hemodialysis. A circuit such as the one shown in Fig. 4.1 should be used to reduce the membrane pressure due to fragility of the plasma filter. The use of a parallel circuit can maintain therapeutic efficacy while reducing the load on the plasma filter. When combining PE with HD (F) in a serial circuit a technician should monitor the procedure and stop it if necessary to prevent overfiltration at the HD (F) side caused by reduced or obstructed blood flow at the PE side.

Hepatic encephalopathy is brain dysfunction that can occur if the liver fails to adequately remove toxic substances from the blood. Alerting influence is reported to remove toxic substances using PE + HD (F).

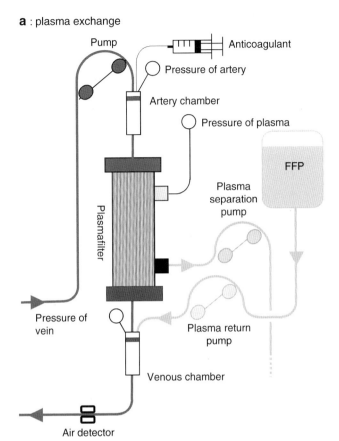

FIGURE 4.1 Circuit of plasma exchange. (**a**) Plasma exchange: separated plasma at the plasma filter is replaced with an equal volume of plasma and albumin. (**b**) PE + HD (serial circuit): plasma replacement is followed by hemodialysis, which is used to remove sodium citrate from FFP and provide renal support. (**c**) PE + HD (parallel/serial circuit): blood separation at the blood removal site reduces the blood flow to the plasma filter

b : PE + HD (series current)

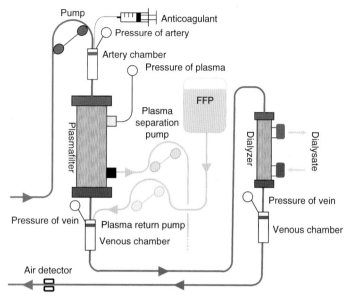

c : PE + HD (parallel/serial circuit)

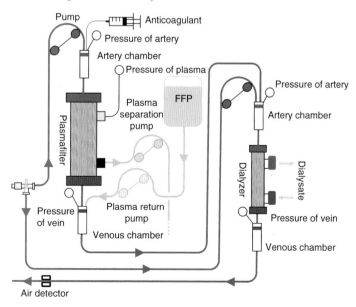

FIGURE 4.1 (continued)

Chapter 5
Double Filtration Plasmapheresis

Daisuke Katagri and Kana Mogi

> **Main Points**
> - The use of two filter membranes with different size pores in double filtration plasmapheresis (DFPP) allows removal of a wider range of toxic substances.
> - Less replacement fluid is needed with DFPP compared with plasma exchange (PE).

5.1 Introduction

Double filtration plasmapheresis (DFPP) is a type of plasma exchange (PE) in which two filters with different pore sizes are used to separate toxic substances from plasma. The

D. Katagri (✉)
Department of Nephrology & Endocrinology, University Hospital,
The University of Tokyo, 7-3-1 Hongo, Bunkyo-ku, Tokyo 113-8655, Japan
e-mail: dkatagiri-tky@umin.ac.jp

K. Mogi
Department of Hemodialysis & Apheresis, University Hospital,
The University of Tokyo, 7-3-1 Hongo, Bunkyo-ku, Tokyo 113-8655, Japan

E. Noiri and N. Hanafusa (eds.), *The Concise Manual of Apheresis Therapy,* DOI 10.1007/978-4-431-54412-8_5,
© Springer Japan 2014

two-stage filtration allows the removal of albumin and its return to the patient's circulation. This feature provides the advantage of reducing the need for replacement fluid and the associated complications, including allergic reaction and infection, that can occur with PE. Using DFPP also reduces the high cost of replacement fluid.

5.2   Basic Principles of DFPP

The DFPP circuit is illustrated in Fig. 5.1. Blood is removed from the patient's circulation via the vascular access and separated into its cellular components and plasma in the plasma separator (first membrane). The plasma then passes through the plasma component separator (second membrane), where fractionation of high and low molecular weight substances takes place. The toxic or pathogenic substances are separated from the plasma and discarded. The cells and other necessary components, including albumin, are returned to the circulation.

5.2.1   Plasma Separator

Commercially available plasma separators have a hollow-fiber membrane with about a 0.3 mm pore size. Because the maximum allowable working pressure varies with different membranes, care should be taken to avoid hemolysis caused by trans-membrane pressure (TMP).

5.2.2   Plasma Component Separator

After filtration in the plasma separator, the plasma is fractionated into large and small molecular weight components in the plasma component separator. High molecular weight components (e.g. IgG, IgA, IgM, C3, C4, fibrinogen, LDL) are discarded. Low molecular weight components, including

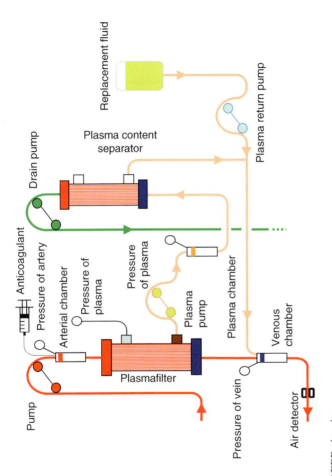

FIGURE 5.1 DFPP circuit

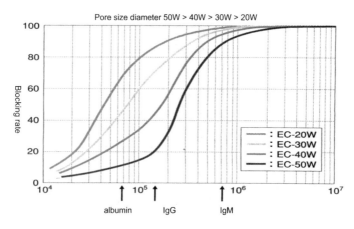

FIGURE 5.2 Molecular weight cut off of the plasma component separator

essential substances such as albumin, are returned to the patient's circulation. A plasma separator that discards the least amount of albumin and the highest amount of pathogenic substances is preferred. A separator with a small pore size is used for removing IgG, whereas a large pore size separator is appropriate for removing IgM or LDL. Figure 5.2 shows the blocking rates achieved according to the molecular weight and micropore diameter of the separator. For more information about commercially available plasma separators and plasma component separators, refer to Chap. 2.

5.2.3 Replacement Fluid

Albumin is commonly used as replacement fluid with DFPP. The risk of infection is lower with albumin than with fresh frozen plasma (FFP). The risk of allergic reaction is also lower with albumin because it does not contain numerous protein antigens. Albumin often is diluted with 5 % dextrose in water when used as replacement fluid. Injection solvent should not be used for the dilution because it may cause severe

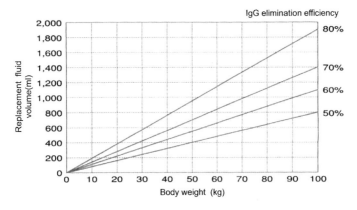

FIGURE 5.3 Quick reference for replacement fluid volume [1]

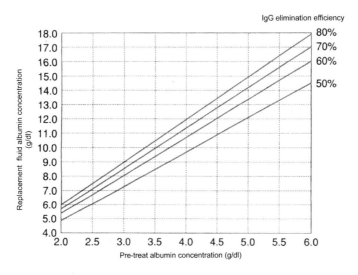

FIGURE 5.4 Quick reference for replacement fluid albumin concentration [1]

hyponatremia and hemolysis. The volume of replacement fluid should equal the volume discarded by the plasma component separator. The replacement fluid volume and albumin concentration were determined as shown in Figs. 5.3 and 5.4 [1].

The method shown in Figs. 5.3 and 5.4 can be used under the following conditions:

1. With the Evaflux 2A® or Cascadeflo EC-20W® plasma component separators.
2. Allow to the point −10 % of patient's circulating blood plasma loss.
3. With a plasma flow rate at the plasma component separator of 25 mL per minute, a filtration flow rate of 20 mL per minute, and a discard/replacement fluid flow rate of 5 mL per minute.

The replacement fluid volume is determined according to the patient's body weight to achieve the IgG elimination efficiency as shown in Fig. 5.3. The albumin concentration of the replacement fluid is determined according to the patient's pretreatment albumin concentration to achieve the IgG elimination efficiency as shown in Fig. 5.4. For example, an albumin concentration three times that of the patient's pretreatment albumin level would be needed to achieve an 80 % IgG elimination efficiency. The volume of the replacement fluid is reduced or eliminated with a plasma component separator with a large pore size that filters more albumin.

5.2.4 Priming

DFPP is primed by a two-stage cleaning procedure. First, the internal side (blood side) of the plasma separator should be gently cleaned, taking care not to damage the hollow fiber. Next, flush the filter with normal saline and clean the pore and external (colature) side of the hollow fiber. Finally, clean the internal and external sides of the plasma component separator.

The fluid level on the external side of the plasma separator should be maintained within the appropriate range as higher levels can cause elevated TMP, resulting in fixture of the colature to the membrane surface. The fluid level should be set to avoid the introduction of air into the plasma component separator. The automated priming function can be used by operators unaccustomed to manual priming.

5.3   Notice During Treatment

The blood flow rate must be faster than 50 mL per minute to avoid coagulation in the circuit. The filtration rate in the plasma separator (first membrane) is about 30 % of the blood flow rate depending on the patient's hematocrit level. Eighty percent of the plasma should be treated in the plasma component separator (second membrane) and the remaining 20 % discarded. The same volume of supplemental fluid is returned to the patient's circulation. The patient's condition and vital signs should be monitored during therapy. The risk of hypotension is increased at the start of treatment and during the administration of replacement fluid. A gradual increase in blood flow rate and filtration rate are effective for preventing hypotension. The inner pressure of the circuit should be monitored to prevent hemolysis and coagulation in the circuit and membrane. If available, a leakage detector should be used on the filtrate side.

Heparin, low molecular weight heparin, and nafamostat mesylate are used for anticoagulation. The activated coagulation time (ACT) should be monitored because of the frequently long duration of extracorporeal circulation and should be within 180–220 s if heparin is used. Several clotting factors are eliminated with DFPP. The heparin dose must be adjusted according to the ACT during each treatment session. Nafamostat mesylate is used for patients in whom heparin is contraindicated.

5.4   Notice at the Completion of Therapy

The patient's condition and vital signs should be monitored at the end of therapy and at the start of blood and plasma return. Two methods can be used to return treated blood to the circulation: (a) the blood cells are returned to the vein chamber, followed by the plasma, or (b) the plasma is returned with air, followed by the blood cells Either normal saline or air can be used for blood return. Normal saline is safer than air, but may result in volume overload.

5.5   Adverse Effects

5.5.1   *Allergic Reaction and Anaphylaxis*

Allergic reaction and anaphylaxis have been reported with the use of blood derivatives, although the frequency is less than 0.1 %. In most cases, symptoms develop within 10 min after starting administration. In such cases, therapy should be discontinued and appropriate measures taken.

5.5.2   *Symptoms due to Decreasing Colloid Oncotic Pressure*

Hypotension may occur in some situations, even though the replacement fluid volume or albumin concentration were appropriately determined. If hypotension occurs, additional albumin should be given or the fluid replacement rate increased if the volume of circulating blood is decreased according to measurement with a device such as CRIT-LINE™.

Reference

1. Eguchi K (2007) How to use replacement fluid and setting of optimum concentration. Ther Apher Dial 26(1):36–47

Chapter 6
Plasma Adsorption

Yasuyuki Watanabe and Maki Tsukamoto

Main Points
- Plasma adsorption can clear the etiologic agent in plasma selectively.
- The risk of infection is low compared with other plasma apheresis treatments because there is no need for blood preparations.

6.1 Introduction

Plasma adsorption is a therapy for clearing an etiologic agent from plasma that has been separated from whole blood through a plasma adsorption device. Depending on the kind of adsorbent, the causative agent can be eliminated selectively. Commonly, the procedure does not need any blood preparation, so there is a low risk of infection. It is often used for autoimmune neuropathy and myopathy.

Y. Watanabe • M. Tsukamoto (✉)
Department of Nephrology and Endocrinology, University Hospital,
The University of Tokyo, 7-3-1 Hongo, Bunkyo-ku, Tokyo 113-8655, Japan
e-mail: mtsukamoto-tky@umin.ac.jp

E. Noiri and N. Hanafusa (eds.), *The Concise Manual of Apheresis Therapy*, DOI 10.1007/978-4-431-54412-8_6,
© Springer Japan 2014

6.2   The Construction of the Dialysis Circuit and Priming

6.2.1   The Construction of the Dialysis Circuit for Plasma Adsorption (Fig. 6.1)

Figure 6.1 indicates the general construction of the circuit for plasma adsorption. The plasma separated from the blood is directed through the plasma adsorption device and the etio-

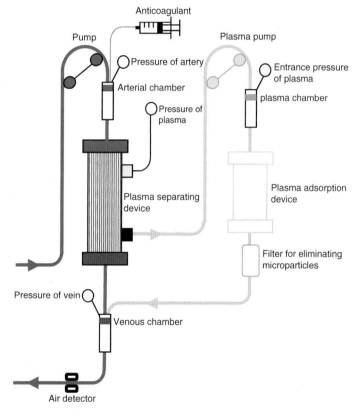

FIGURE 6.1 The circuit of plasma adsorption

logic agent is eliminated selectively. The plasma then returns to the patient through the circuit. To prevent plasma adsorbent from flowing out, a filter for catching minute particles is set behind the plasma adsorption device (Table 6.1).

6.2.2   The Construction of the Plasma Adsorption Column and the Principle of Adsorption

The plasma adsorbent consists of a ligand that has an affinity for the etiology agent and a supporting carrier. The ligand has the ability to selectively bind the substance to be adsorbed and the carrier supports the ligand and has an ability to change the adsorptive specificity within each column according to molecular weight. Adsorptive devices can be divided into two groups depending on the adsorption mechanism used: hydrophobic or electrostatic interaction (see Sect. 1.1 in Chap. 1).

6.2.3   Priming

Priming is divided into two processes: rinsing the plasma separating device and rinsing the adsorption device. The priming process is a little different for each device. One method is to rinse the plasma side of the plasma adsorption device after rinsing the blood side of the plasma separating device (Fig. 6.2). In this method, the priming solution flows in the same direction as the plasma. Another method is to rinse the plasma separating device and the adsorption device separately (Fig. 6.3). In this method, connectors are used so that the priming solution flows in the opposite direction through the plasma adsorption device. For both methods, care must be taken to not mix air into the adsorption device. The connectors should be attached after eliminating air near the port. The plasma separating device is a fragile membrane, so excessive impact or pressure should be avoided to prevent damage.

TABLE 6.1 The characteristics of each plasma adsorption device

Ligand		Name	Force	Object substance	Content for filling (mL)	Solution for filling	Priming volume (mL)
Hydrophobic amino acid	Phenylalanine	Immusorba PH-350	Hydrophobic interaction	Rheumatoid factor, immune complex, anti-DNA antibody	350	Saline	300
	Tryptophan	Immusorba TR-350	Hydrophobic interaction	Anti-acetylcholine receptor antibody	350	0.01 % disodium pyrosulfite	300
Dextran sulfate		Liposorber LA-15	Electrostatic interaction	LDL	150	Solution of citric acid and sodium citrate	140
		Liposorber LA-40S	Electrostatic interaction	LDL	400	Solution of citric acid and sodium citrate	370

Styrene divinyl benzene copolymer	Selesorb	Electrostatic interaction	Anti-cardiolipin antibody, immune complex	150	Solution of citric acid and sodium citrate	140
	Plasorba BRS-350	Electrostatic interaction	Bilirubin, bile acid	110	Pyrogen-free solution	300
	Medisorba BL-300	Electrostatic interaction	Bilirubin, bile acid	110	Pyrogen-free solution	300

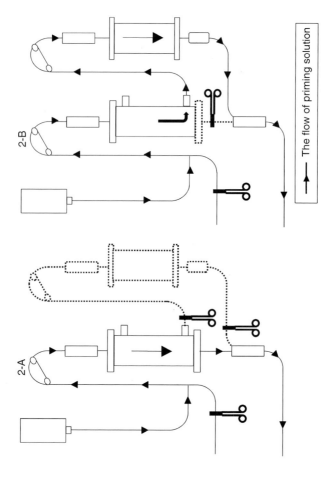

FIGURE 6.2 A method for priming and rinsing that follows the normal course of the circuit

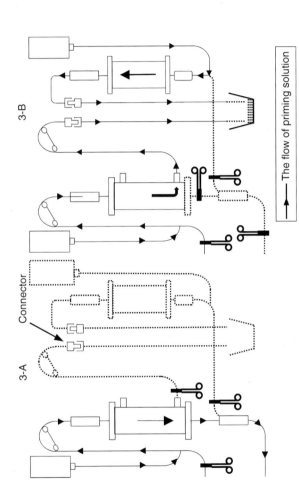

3-B

3-A

Connector

→ The flow of priming solution

FIGURE 6.3   A method for priming and rinsing that uses connectors to route the priming fluid through the adsorption device in the opposite direction as the plasma flow

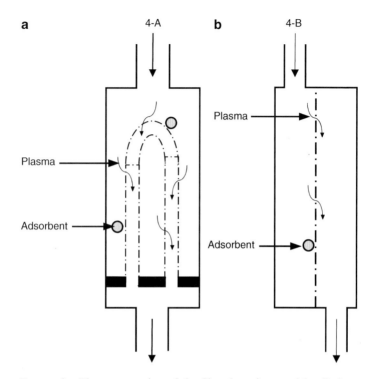

FIGURE 6.4 The construction of the filter for microparticle elimination (**a**) with hollow fiber (**b**) with partition

The filters for eliminating minute particles use one of two filtration methods: hollow fiber (Fig. 6.4a) or partitioned (Fig. 6.4b). It is difficult to eliminate air after the membrane has become wet from priming, so much care should be taken to prevent air from entering.

6.2.4   Anticoagulant

In plasma adsorption the duration of extracorporeal circulation is long and an anticoagulant is needed; heparin and nafamostat mesylate are often used. Regulation of the dose and monitoring of the activated coagulation time (ACT) is needed, and it should be noted that nafamostat mesylate has the effect of inhibiting the production of bradykinin.

6.3 Points to Note

6.3.1 From the Start of and During Treatment

When extracorporeal circulation is started, blood flow should be increased gradually to guard against a decrease in blood pressure. At the same time, care should be taken to confirm the condition of the blood removal and to check if there are any rapid increases of pressure in the circuits.

The velocity of the separated plasma should be increased gradually while monitoring the change in circulation. Commonly, the velocity of the separated plasma should not be greater than 30 % of the blood flow.

Monitoring patient blood pressure carefully is important because a rapid decrease of blood pressure is often seen when the returned plasma and blood enters the body after passing through the plasma adsorption device.

The transmembrane pressure of the plasma separating device is related to the degree of coagulation for the separating membrane and the pressure at the entrance of the adsorption device is related to the degree of coagulation within the adsorption device. Care should be taken to ensure proper anticoagulation and monitoring of these areas.

6.3.2 Retransfusion

During retransfusion, circulating blood volume increases rapidly in a short time, and care should be taken to monitor this change. The retransfusion procedure is different for each device. One method of retransfusion starts at the blood side, followed by the plasma side, and another starts at the plasma side, utilizing air, followed by the blood side. Columns using amino acids as ligands require retransfusion with air, because desorption would occur if saline were used. Throughout this procedure, it is important to not allow air to enter the body.

6.3.3   Anaphylactic Shock Induced by the Inhibitor of Angiotensin Converting Enzyme

If a negative charge is used in the process, bradykinin levels can rise during plasma adsorption. Kininase II, an angiotensin-converting enzyme, usually resolves this issue. However, use of an inhibitor of angiotensin-converting enzymes (ACE-I) would block kininase, allowing the concentration of bradykinin to increase, possibly resulting in anaphylactic shock. This is why the use of ACE-Is is prohibited with TR-350, LA 40S, LA-15, and Selesorb adsorption devices.

6.4   The Characteristics of Particular Adsorption Devices and Points to Be Noted

6.4.1   Columns with Hydrophobic Amino Acid (Phenylalanine, Tryptophan)

6.4.1.1   Immusorba TR-350

These columns use tryptophan as a ligand that selectively adsorbs through hydrophobic interactions and eliminates autoantibodies, like immune complexes or anti-acetylcholine receptor antibodies. The efficiency of the adsorption is different for each IgG subclass. IgG_4 tends to de-adsorb easily compared with the other IgG subclasses, and the desorption of IgG_4 starts after processing 1 L of plasma. The TR-350 has very strong hydrophobic interactions, and can adsorb anti-acetylcholine receptor antibodies with three times stronger affinity than can the PH-350. However, it also adsorbs fibrinogen. Because frequent treatments in a short time can cause a decrease in this protein, fibrinogen levels should be monitored. It has also been reported that a sudden decrease of blood pressure occurs after processing 1.2–1.5 L of plasma because of the increased concentration of bradykinin.

6.4.1.2 Immusorba PH-350

This column uses phenylalanine as a ligand that selectively adsorbs through hydrophobic interactions and eliminates immune complexes, anti-DNA antibodies, and rheumatoid factors.

6.4.1.3 Points to Note

Plasma flow should be set to less than 20 mL/ min to prevent a reduction in blood pressure. Air is used at the time of retransfusion, because desorption would occur if saline were used, however, throughout this procedure, care must be taken to not allow air to enter the body.

6.4.2 Columns with Dextran Sulfate

Columns using dextran sulfate as a ligand selectively eliminate substances through electrostatic interactions between the negative and positive charges of dextran sulfate.

Changing the bore diameter will change the ability of the column to adsorb a substance. Liposorber (LA-40S, LA-15) columns can eliminate LDL selectively with a large bore diameter. Alternatively, Selesorb can eliminate immune complexes, anti-DNA antibodies, and anti-cardiolipin antibodies better with a small bore diameter.

Hypocalcemia can be induced because both columns also adsorb Ca^{2+} ions. Priming with a transfusion that contains more than 3 mEq/L Ca^{2+} ions can make the column approach its maximum adsorption level for Ca^{2+} ions and prevent hypocalcemia. However, maltose-lactated Ringer's solution is not good for priming.

Liposorber columns (LA-40S, LA-15) can eliminate LDL selectively through their strong electrostatic interactions with apolipoprotein B.

A Liposorber/Selesorb system can be used repeatedly to release LDL, and using this system, the plasma volume can be increased dramatically compared with using a one-column system.

6.4.3   Columns to Adsorb Bilirubin and Bile Acid

6.4.3.1   Plasorba BRS-350 and Medisorba BL-300

These columns use a styrene-divinyl benzene copolymer, which is an ion exchange resin, as a ligand that selectively eliminates negatively charged bilirubin and bile acid. The plasma flow should be set to less than 20 mL per minute to prevent a reduction in blood pressure.

A filter for eliminating microparticles is not necessary for this column, because coating the ligand with a hydroxyl-ethyl-methacrylate copolymer (poly-HEMA) and using a non-woven fabric incorporated into the exit of the adsorption device prevents microparticles from flowing out.

However, more saline with heparin is necessary for priming and anticoagulation during treatment, because the column also adsorbs the negatively charged heparin.

References

1. Nakazono K (2007) Rinsho Touseki 23:48–55
2. Iwamoto H, Koga N (1999) Jituyo Ketuekijouka Ryoho 77–83

Chapter 7
Cryofiltration

Daisuke Katagiri and Hiroko Yamamoto

Main Points
- Cryofiltration is a modification of double filtration plasmapheresis (DFPP) that involves cooling the separated plasma.
- Cryofiltration is based on the formation of cryoglobulin or cryogel upon cooling of pathogenic proteins in plasma.

7.1 Concept

Cryofiltration is a modification of DFPP that involves cooling the separated plasma at the plasma separator (first membrane) to gelatinize the proteins in the plasma, which are then ablated at

D. Katagiri (✉)
Department of Nephrology & Endocrinology, University Hospital,
The University of Tokyo, 7-3-1 Hongo, Bunkyo-ku,
Tokyo 113-8655, Japan
e-mail: dkatagiri-tky@umin.ac.jp

H. Yamamoto
Department of Hemodialysis & Apheresis, University Hospital,
The University of Tokyo, 7-3-1 Hongo, Bunkyo-ku,
Tokyo 113-8655, Japan

E. Noiri and N. Hanafusa (eds.), *The Concise Manual of Apheresis Therapy*, DOI 10.1007/978-4-431-54412-8_7, © Springer Japan 2014

the large pore plasma component separator (second membrane).

The gelatinized and ablated proteins form into cryoglobulin or cryogel. Cryoglobulin is the collective term for abnormal proteins, including single immunoglobulins and multi-immunoglobulins (mainly IgG or IgM), that clump into a gel at 39.2 °F and dissolve at 98.6 °F. Cryogel is a complex of heparin, fibronectin, and fibrinogen. Fibronectin and fibrinogen precipitate with cooling and gelatinize with high affinity to heparin. EDA + fibronectin is important for the formation of cryogel with an affinity to heparin [1].

7.2   Treatment of Cryoglobulinemia

Cryofiltration is used to treat patients with cryoglobulinemia, a medical condition in which the blood contains large amounts of cryoglobulins. Patients may have essential cryoglobulinemia or secondary cryoglobulinemia associated with various diseases, including macroglobulinemia, multiple myeloma, connective tissue disease, and hepatitis C infection. The cryoglobulin test is used to make the diagnosis in patients with purpura, Raynaud's phenomenon, or the earlier mentioned conditions [2]. Patients with autoimmune diseases such as rheumatoid arthritis or systemic lupus erythematosus, or patients with EDA + fibronectin—rich, such as multiple myeloma may also be treated with cryofiltration to eliminate autoantibody or immune complex, which precipitates as cryogel. Because only patients with cryoglobulinemia are treated with cryofiltration in our hospital, this chapter will primarily address this indication.

7.3   Methods

The cryofiltration circuit, illustrated in Fig. 7.1, is similar to the circuit used for DFPP. The differences between the two types of circuits are described later.

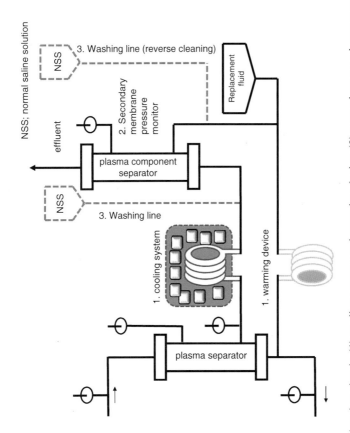

FIGURE 7.1 Cryofiltration circuit. (**1**) cooling system and warming device. (**2**) secondary membrane pressure monitoring. (**3**) line for washing secondary membrane

7.3.1   Cooling System and Warming Device
[Fig. 7.1 (1)]

The cryofiltration circuit incorporates a cooling system, which cools the plasma with iced water, cold air, or a cooling plate. Iced water cooling is an easy-to-use technique that does not require a dedicated cooling device for cryofiltration. A cooling compartment connected to the circuit contains a coiled tube immersed in iced water that is kept at a temperature of about 39.2 °F (32–50 °F). An artificial heart-lung machine can be used to easily control the temperature. After the cryoglobulin or cryogel is separated from the plasma, the plasma is rewarmed to about 98.6 °F with a warming device attached to the circuit. If warming is inadequate, use of a second warming device should be considered.

7.3.2   Secondary Membrane Pressure Monitoring
[Fig. 7.1 (2)]

The plasma component separator membrane may become clogged by precipitated cryoglobulin or cryogel. Therefore, it is important to monitor the pressure of this membrane. Elevated pressure is an indication that the membrane should be washed to clear the pores of any cryoglobulin or cryogel.

7.3.3   Line for Washing Secondary Membrane
[Fig. 7.1 (3)]

The secondary membrane can be washed with a small amount of separated plasma if the pressure becomes elevated. Normal saline should be used in cases with frequently elevated pressure. Washing may be performed from the inner to the outer side or from the outer to the inner side of the secondary membrane. A line for washing with normal saline can be connected to the circuit as shown in the figure. If a dedicated washing device is not available, the washing procedure should be adjusted for manual operation.

7.4   Points to Note

In our hospital, the EC-50W/Evaflux 5A plasma component membrane (second membrane) is used for cryofiltration. Replacement fluid generally is not needed for this application; however, hypoalbuminemia or clotting factor deficiency may occur with multiple washings of the secondary membrane. Changes in blood volume should be monitored with the Crit-Line In-Line Monitor™ [In-Line Diagnostics, Kaysville, UT] device during the procedure, and replacement of albumin should also be considered. If severe clotting factor deficiency occurs, replacement clotting factor should be administered or the procedure terminated. If a different type of plasma component membrane is used, replacement fluid will be needed as with DFPP. Refer to Chap. 5 for information on replacement fluid parameters.

7.5   Clinical Effect

The expected benefits of cryofiltration include improvements in circulatory disorders such as Raynaud's disease and purpura and immune-complex diseases such as nephritis, arthralgia, and peripheral neuropathy.

7.6   Comparison with Other Treatments

If a dedicated device for cryofiltration is not available, it should be difficult to attempt this procedure. However it is more complicated than DFPP, cryofiltration has the advantage of eliminating cryoglobulin without the need for scarce blood products.

References

1. Yonekawa M (2002) Practical cooling plasma filtration. Ther Apher Dial 21(2):156–158
2. Sugisaki T (2001) Diverseness and detecting method of cryo-globulin. Med Technol 29(7):709–712

Chapter 8
Double Filtration Plasmapheresis Thermo-Mode (DF Thermo)

Mizuki Yamano

> **Main Points**
> - DF thermo is a type of double filtration plasma-pheresis (DFPP) that does not require fluid replacement when a large pore size plasma component membrane is used.
> - Heating increases the plasma processing volume and maintains or improves the sieving coefficient (verified by in vitro experimentation).

8.1 Double Filtration Plasmapheresis Thermo-Mode (DF Thermo)

DF thermo is a type of double filtration plasmapheresis (DFPP) with the following characteristics: (1) the plasma component membrane (second filter) has a large pore size

M. Yamano (✉)
Department of Hemodialysis & Apheresis, University Hospital, The
University of Tokyo, 7-3-1 Hongo, Bunkyo-ku, Tokyo 113-8655, Japan
e-mail: mizukiymn@yahoo.co.jp

E. Noiri and N. Hanafusa (eds.), *The Concise Manual
of Apheresis Therapy*, DOI 10.1007/978-4-431-54412-8_8,
© Springer Japan 2014

with a high sieving coefficient for albumin (Evaflux® 5A: Kawasumi Laboratories Inc., Cascade Flow® EC-50W: Asahi Kasei Kuraray Medical), (2) replacement fluid (blood product) is not necessary with DF thermo, (3) fractionation and separation are performed after heating the plasma components with a heating unit added to the recirculation circuit. This method increases the total plasma processing volume, improving fractionation performance [1] and (4) the plasma recirculation system eliminates the production of waste fluid and helps control infections.

8.2   The Effect of Warming

The plasma in the recirculation circuit is controlled at a constant temperature. Filtering plasma through the plasma component membrane at room temperature reduces the plasma temperature to about 86 °F, resulting in increased plasma viscosity. Increased plasma viscosity reduces the performance of plasma fractionation. With DF thermo, warming the plasma to 108 °F maintains the performance of plasma fractionation at a high level.

8.3   Circuit Configuration

The circuit configuration used for DF thermo is similar to that used for the DFPP circuit, with some modifications (Fig. 8.1). Blood removed from the patient is directed to the plasma separator, where it is separated into the blood cell and plasma components. The plasma component is then introduced into the plasma component membrane and further separated mainly into the albumin-globulin fraction and the lipid fraction. The albumin fraction (molecular weight ~69,000 Da), most of which is filtered by the plasma component membrane, is returned to the circulation together with

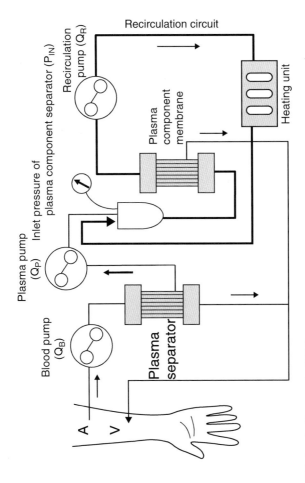

FIGURE 8.1 DF circuit diagram in DF thermo

the separated blood components. However, because LDL has a molecular weight of 2,000–3,000 kDa, it is not filtered by the plasma component membrane. It is derived by a recirculation pump, and continuously run through the recirculation circuit shown by the bold line in Fig. 8.1 and does not return to the blood stream.

8.4 Selection of Plasma Component Membrane

For specifications, refer to Chap. 5. The plasma component membrane used for DFPP is selected for the specific disease or target substance to be removed and the treatment parameters are determined accordingly. In other words, it is necessary to use a fractionator designed specifically for the fraction to be removed. DF thermo often is used to remove the IgM fraction (molecular weight about 950 kDa), the LDL fraction (molecular weight about 1,300 kDa), and viruses with a higher molecular weight. The sieving coefficient for albumin is low with use of a relatively small pore membrane, resulting in a need for fluid replacement with a blood product such as albumin solution. Alternatively, the sieving coefficient for albumin is high with the use of a large pore size membrane; hence, replacement fluid is not necessary.

8.5 Equipment and Features Required for DF Thermo

The KM-9000, KPS-8800Ce (Kawasumi Laboratories Inc.) is used for DF thermo. The latest device has self-priming, automatic blood return, and guidance functions, so it provides user-friendliness. DF thermo requires the use of three pumps: a blood pump, a plasma separation pump, and a recirculation pump.

8.6 Setting the Operating Parameters and Monitoring

Table 8.1 shows the typical operating conditions for DF thermo.

The pressure and the transmembrane pressure (TMP) are monitored during therapy. Increased pressure at the venous or arterial side indicates thrombosis in the blood circuit and plasma separator. An increase in the inlet pressure of the plasma component membrane indicates thrombosis in the plasma circuit and plasma component membrane. Increased TMP in the plasma separator indicates reduced filtration caused by a clogged membrane. Because plasma separation at excessively high TMP leads to hemolysis, monitoring the TMP is very important. According to the equipment package insert, TMP must be maintained at less than 60 mmHg. Monitoring the TMP at the plasma component membrane is important because it allows early detection of poor fractionation performance and prediction of albumin loss.

TABLE 8.1 General operating conditions for DF thermo

Plasma separator (first filter)	OP-05/08W, PE-05/08, FS-05/08
Plasma component membrane (second filter)	Evaflux 5A, Cascadeflo EC-50W
Blood pump (Q_B)	80–120 mL/min (depends on vascular access)
Plasma separator pump (Q_P)	20–30 mL/min (depends on vascular access)
Recirculation pump (Q_P)	20 or 80 mL/min (fixed value for each device)
Inlet pressure of plasma component membrane (P_{IN})	Below 500 mmHg
Plasma processing volume	3,000–4,000 mL (depends on the patient physique)

8.7   Replacement Fluid

Fluid replacement generally is not needed when using a plasma component membrane with a high sieving coefficient for albumin (e.g., Evaflux-5A, Cascade Flow EC-50W).

8.8   Indication Diseases, Indicators of Treatment, and Frequency of Therapy

Table 8.2 shows indications for DF thermo and the recommended treatment frequency for each.

8.9   Anticoagulant Therapy

The indication for anticoagulant therapy with DF thermo treatment is similar to that used with DFPP and plasma exchange (PE).

Heparin generally is used for patients who do not have a bleeding tendency. The dose should be adjusted according to the patient's physique and condition. As a guide, the initial dose ranges from 1,000 to 2,000 IU and the continuous dose is 1,000–2,000 IU/h to maintain an activated coagulation time (ACT) of 150–200 s.

Low molecular weight heparin is often used for patients with a mild bleeding tendency. The dose of low molecular weight heparin generally is one-half the dose of heparin due to the longer half-life of low molecular weight heparin.

Patients with a severe bleeding tendency often are treated with nafamostat mesylate administered as a continuous dose of 20–40 mg/h. The dosage should be adjusted according to the severity of the patient's bleeding.

The following points should be considered when selecting anticoagulant therapy. Repeated treatments with DF thermo results in removal of some coagulation factors, particularly fibrinogen. Therefore, if the time to hemostasis is prolonged due to hypofibrinogenemia, switching to another anticoagulant such as nafamostat mesylate should be considered.

TABLE 8.2 Indications for DF Thermo

Indications	Details of the indication	Recommended frequency of treatment
Familial hypercholesterolemia	Patients exhibiting one of the following criteria concurrent with xanthoma, in whom coronary arteriosclerosis has been diagnosed by stress electrocardiogram and coronary angiography. 1. Homozygous for hypercholesterolemia with serum total cholesterol >500 mg/dL during a stable fasting period. 2. Heterozygous for hypercholesterolemia with serum total cholesterol >400 mg/dL while on diet therapy (maintaining stable body weight and serum albumin level), and with serum cholesterol ^{3}250 mg/dL after pharmacotherapy.	Once a week as maintenance therapy
Arteriosclerotic obliteration	Patients with all of the following criteria. 1. Fontaine classification II, III, or IV 2. Hypercholesterolemia with serum total cholesterol >220 mg/dL or LDL cholesterol >140 mg/dL after pharmacotherapy. 3. Inoperable peripheral arterial disease (PAD) (e.g., arterial obstruction of popliteal or peripheral side) that cannot be adequately treated with conventional medical therapies.	Limited to sequential treatments 10 times/3 months

(continued)

TABLE 8.2 (continued)

Indications	Details of the indication	Recommended frequency of treatment
Chronic hepatitis C	Patients with HCV genotype II (1b) serum RNA level >100 KIU/mL immediately after interferon therapy.	Limited to five times as preconditioning for interferon therapy
Focal segmental glomerulosclerosis	Patients whose condition has not resolved with conventional pharmacotherapy, with nephrotic status, and serum cholesterol level >250 mg/dL.	Limited to sequential treatments 10 times/3 months
Macroglobulinemia		Limited to sequential treatments once a week/3 months

8.10   Points to Note

Compared with hemodialysis, DFPP has a long circuit configuration consisting of two modules (a blood side circuit and a plasma side circuit). The priming volume is large, consisting of approximately 400 mL. Therefore, caution must be taken to avoid a drop in blood pressure due to hemodilution when treating children and patients of small physical size. Hypoalbuminemia due to the lower recovery rate of albumin in a plasma component membrane can decrease the colloid oncotic pressure, leading to a drop in blood pressure.

Hemodynamic status, including blood pressure and pulse, should be monitored during treatment and appropriate measures should be taken in the case of a change in status.

Although rare, allergic reactions to medical materials or anticoagulants may occur. Therefore, it is important to monitor the patient's vital signs and condition to detect any change in respiratory status, body temperature, or state of consciousness and possible symptoms such as skin rash or itching.

The potential for albumin loss and IgM removal are issues with DF thermo [2]. Patients treated with repeated DF thermo should be monitored for such losses.

References

1. Taketoshi N et al (1995) Jpn J Apher 13(Suppl):74
2. Konno Y et al (2005) Jpn J Apher 24(1):91–98

Chapter 9
Plasma Diafiltration

Hajime Nakae

Main Points

- Plasma diafiltration (PDF) is a blood-purification therapy in which simple plasma exchange (PE) is performed using a selective membrane plasma separator (sieving coefficient for albumin, 0.3), while the dialysate flows outside the plasma separator.
- PDF can remove both water-soluble and albumin-bound substances.
- Coagulation factors are preserved because this membrane has a sieving coefficient of 0 for fibrinogen and immunoglobulin M.
- PDF is useful for patients with acute liver failure, severe sepsis, acute pancreatitis, or intoxication.

H. Nakae (✉)
Department of Emergency and Critical Care Medicine, Akita University
Graduate School of Medicine, 1-1-1 Hondo, Akita 010-8543, Japan
e-mail: nakaeh@doc.med.akita-u.ac.jp

E. Noiri and N. Hanafusa (eds.), *The Concise Manual*
of Apheresis Therapy, DOI 10.1007/978-4-431-54412-8_9,
© Springer Japan 2014

9.1   Introduction

Acute liver failure can cause various toxins to circulate in the bloodstream. To remove these toxins, several kinds of artificial liver support systems (ALSSs) can be used, such as plasma exchange (PE), high-flow hemodialysis (HD), high-volume hemofiltration (HF), high-flow volume hemodiafiltration (HDF), and albumin dialysis therapies. Plasma diafiltration (PDF) is a blood-purification therapy in which simple PE is performed using a selective membrane plasma separator while the dialysate flows outside the hollow fibers of the plasma separator [1–4]. This method is a useful ALSS for the removal of both water-soluble and albumin-bound toxins, and has a reasonable cost.

9.2   PDF Procedures

9.2.1   Flow

Simple PE is performed with a membrane plasma separator [Evacure EC-2A plasma separator (Kawasumi Laboratories Inc., Tokyo, Japan)] while the dialysate flows outside the plasma separator; HDF is performed simultaneously. A blood flow rate of 80–100 mL/min is used. Dialysate is circulated through the plasma separator at a flow rate of 1,500 mL/h, and additional replacement volume is provided to the patient at a flow rate of 690 mL/h. Fluid removal is performed by reducing the replacement flow rate to 450 mL/h at most. In addition, a 1,200 mL volume of normal fresh frozen plasma (FFP) and 50 mL of 25 % albumin solution is intravenously infused over an 8-h period (Fig. 9.1).

9.2.2   Features

The Evacure EC-2A plasma separator has a pore size of 0.01 mm, which is much smaller than that of conventional

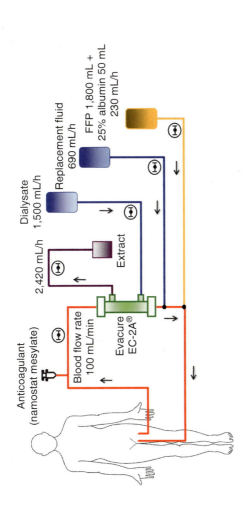

Figure 9.1 Schematic representation of PDF. PDF is performed for 8 h once a day as a single session or for 24 h continuously in three sessions, according to the patient's condition. PDF is a simpler modality than plasma exchange with continuous hemodiafiltration (CHDF) and uses only one plasma separator. *FFP* fresh frozen plasma

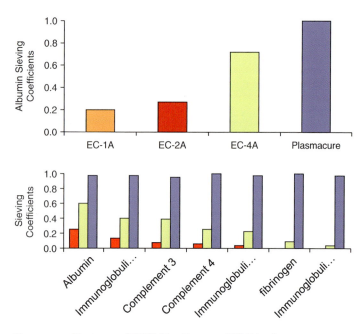

FIGURE 9.2 Features of PDF. The Evacure EC-2A plasma separator
used for PDF has a pore size of 0.01 mm, which is much smaller than
that of standard plasma-separation membranes. This membrane can
selectively remove low and intermediate molecular weight albumin-
bound substances while retaining high molecular weight proteins
such as fibrinogen and immunoglobulin M

plasma separation membranes (0.2–0.4 mm). This ethylene-vinyl
alcohol copolymer membrane has a sieving coefficient of 0.3
for albumin and can thus selectively remove low and intermediate molecular weight albumin-bound substances. In addition, coagulation factors are preserved because this membrane
has a sieving coefficient of 0 for fibrinogen and immunoglobulin M (Fig. 9.2). During PE, it is difficult to completely
control increases in citrate concentrations by administering
FFP. In PDF, the increase in citrate concentration is inhibited
more effectively because smaller amounts of FFP are required
and because HDF is performed simultaneously. Furthermore,
the use of smaller amounts of FFP reduces medical costs

TABLE 9.1 Problems of plasma exchange

Requires large amounts of FFP	Large citrate transfusion • Hypernatremia, hypocalcemia, metabolic alkalosis • Citrate intoxication, nausea, vomiting, convulsion, liver dysfunction Anaphylactic reaction, hypersensitivity Decreased osmotic pressure of plasma colloids • Pulmonary edema, brain edema
Removal of high molecular weight proteins	Loss of essential substances such as clotting factors, a number of hormones

FFP fresh frozen plasma

TABLE 9.2 Comparisons among PDF, PE+CHDF, and MARS®

Variable	PDF	PE+CHDF	MARS®
Circuit	Simple	Complicated	More complicated
FFP (mL/day)	1,800	3,200–4,000	None
Citrate increase	Slight	Moderate	None
Bilirubin removal	Moderate	Good	Moderate
Fibrinogen retention	Good	Poor	Good
Material cost (/procedure)	Low	Middle	High

PDF plasma diafiltration, *PE* plasma exchange, *CHDF* continuous hemodiafiltration, *MARS* molecular adsorbent recirculating system, *FFP* fresh frozen plasma

(Tables 9.1 and 9.2). Excessive amounts of both water-soluble and albumin-bound substances, such as cystatin C, bilirubin, interleukin (IL)-6, and IL-18 can be reduced by PDF [3, 4]. The clearance rate for creatinine and blood urea nitrogen (BUN) is 20 mL/min, and that for cytokines, such as IL-6 and IL-8, is 18 mL/min. Thus, the cytokine sieving coefficient is 0.8–0.9. The concept behind PDF is that dialysis is also performed during this type of selective plasma filtration (Fig. 9.3).

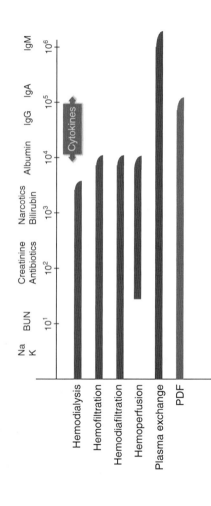

FIGURE 9.3 PDF compared with other blood-purification therapies. Excessive amounts of both water-soluble and albumin-bound substances, such as potassium, bilirubin, and cytokines can be reduced by PDF. *Na* sodium, *K* potassium, *BUN* blood urea nitrogen, *Ig* immunoglobulin

9.2.3   Priming

The blood circuit is flushed with 1,000 mL of heparinized saline.

9.2.4   Anticoagulation

Nafamostat mesylate is administered at an initial dose of 30 mg/h and the concentration is adjusted to maintain an activated coagulation time of 150–180 s.

9.2.5   PDF Session

PDF is performed for 8 h once a day as a single session. Albumin levels did not change significantly on performing PDF for previous studies, but nevertheless, 50 mL of 25 % albumin solution is added at the end of the PDF, to adjust for the loss of albumin by diffusion.

9.3   Options for PDF

9.3.1   Hepatorenal Syndrome

Continuous HD is performed using a PDF circuit. The dialysate flow rate is set to 600 mL/h; 50 mL of 25 % albumin solution is also infused every 8 h, to account for the loss of albumin by diffusion.

9.3.2   Severe Liver Failure

PDF can be performed for 24 h continuously, according to the patient's condition.

9.3.3   Sepsis and Severe Acute Pancreatitis

A patient without disseminated intravascular coagulation (DIC) or bleeding tendency does not need clotting factor-replacement therapy. In such situations, PDF can be performed with a 5 % albumin solution instead of FFP.

9.3.4   Acute Intoxication

Almost all intoxicating substances bind to proteins. PDF is performed to remove the intoxicating substances that have high albumin-binding rates [5].

Note: Outcome from PDF/the MELD Score

According to prospective and multicenter studies examining the use of PDF in patients with acute liver failure, no remarkable differences in prognosis were observed compared to the outcomes from studies using albumin dialysis [6–9]. MARS® and Prometheus® have been considered as bridge therapies for liver transplantation in previous studies. However, PDF was intended to be a direct treatment for acute liver failure, considering the scarcity of donor organs in Japan. Therefore, the number of severe cases, with model for endstage liver disease (MELD) scores of ≥ 40, was larger in the PDF studies than in the MARS® studies.

The MELD score is predictive of survival and is used to prioritize patients with chronic liver disease for orthotopic liver transplantation [10]. This score is also considered to reflect the prognosis for fulminant hepatic failure [11]. The survival rate at a MELD score of ≤ 9 is more than 90 %. The mortality rate at MELD scores of ≥ 40 is ≥ 80 %, but is not considered to be indicative of the need for liver transplantation. In Japan, PDF is recommended for patients with a MELD score of 19, which is indicative of the need for liver transplantation.

References

1. Nakae H, Igarashi T, Tajimi K et al (2007) A case report of hepatorenal syndrome treated with plasma diafiltration (selective plasma filtration with dialysis). Ther Apher Dial 11:391–395
2. Nakae H, Igarashi T, Tajimi K et al (2008) A case of pediatric fulminant hepatitis treated with plasma diafiltration. Ther Apher Dial 12:329–332
3. Nakae H, Eguchi Y, Saotome T et al (2010) Multicenter study of plasma diafiltration in patients with acute liver failure. Ther Apher Dial 14:444–450
4. Nakae H, Eguchi Y, Yoshioka T et al (2011) Plasma diafiltration therapy in patients with postoperative liver failure. Ther Apher Dial 15:406–410
5. Nakae H (2010) Blood purification for intoxication. Contrib Nephrol 166:93–99
6. Evenepoel P, Laleman W, Wilmer A et al (2006) Prometheus versus molecular adsorbents recirculating system: comparison of efficiency in two different liver detoxification devices. Artif Organs 30:276–284
7. Faenza S, Baraldi O, Bernardi M et al (2008) MARS and prometheus: our clinical experience in acute chronic liver failure. Transplant Proc 40:1169–1171
8. Dethloff T, Tofteng F, Frederiksen HJ et al (2008) Effect of prometheus liver assist system on systemic hemodynamics in patients with cirrhosis: a randomized controlled study. World J Gastroenterol 14:2065–2071
9. Grodzicki M, Kotulski M, Leonowicz D et al (2009) Results of treatment of acute liver failure patients with use of the prometheus FPSA system. Transplant Proc 41:3079–3081
10. Kamath PS, Wiesner RH, Malinchoc M et al (2001) A model to predict survival in patients with end-stage liver disease. Hepatology 33:464–470
11. Dhiman RK, Jain S, Maheshwari U et al (2007) Early indicators of prognosis in fulminant hepatic failure: an assessment of the Model for End-Stage Liver Disease (MELD) and King's College Hospital criteria. Liver Transpl 13:814–821

Chapter 10
Direct Plasma Adsorption

Mayumi Miwa and Maki Tsukamoto

Main Points
- Direct plasma adsorption eliminates the targeted substances in the blood by passing the blood through the column directly.
- The device is simple and does not require any dialysate or refilling fluid.
- Carbon adsorption is used for drug intoxication, PMX-DHP is used for sepsis induced by gram-negative rods, and β2 microglobulin adsorption is used for dialysis-related amyloidosis.

M. Miwa • M. Tsukamoto (✉)
Department of Nephrology and Endocrinology, University Hospital,
The University of Tokyo, 7-3-1 Hongo, Bunkyo-ku, Tokyo 113-8655, Japan
e-mail: mtsukamoto-tky@umin.ac.jp

E. Noiri and N. Hanafusa (eds.), *The Concise Manual
of Apheresis Therapy*, DOI 10.1007/978-4-431-54412-8_10,
© Springer Japan 2014

10.1   Direct Plasma Adsorption

Direct plasma adsorption is a method for eliminating pathogenic agents or toxic substances in the blood by perfusion of the blood through the adsorbent material. Adsorption columns are customized for specific target diseases and substances to be eliminated. The three types of adsorption columns are carbon adsorption, PMX-DHP, and b2 microglobulin columns (Table 10.1). Figure 10.1a is an illustration of the adsorption column circuit and Fig. 10.1b shows the combination of a hemoperfusion adsorption column and hemodialysis circuit.

10.2   Important Principles for Hemoperfusion

10.2.1   Rinsing and Priming

The column should be set up so blood flows in the direction of the arrow on the surface of the column. The circuit is rinsed as it is in hemodialysis.

10.2.2   At the Start of and During Therapy

At the start of therapy, the blood flow should be increased gradually until the target flow rate is achieved. The patient's vital signs and functioning of the circuit should be monitored (Fig. 10.2).

The pressure at the entrance and exit of the adsorption device should be monitored throughout the procedure. If the pressure increases to more than 300 mmHg or increases suddenly, the possibility of a clot in the column should be considered.

The blood flow rate should be decreased or therapy stopped if the patient develops any circulatory problems.

The circuit and the patient should be warmed if necessary to prevent a decrease in the patient's body temperature.

TABLE 10.1 Characteristics of types of hemoperfusion

Type of hemoperfusion	Carbon adsorption	Endotoxin adsorption	β2 microglobulin adsorption
Commercial name	DHP-1/Hemosorber CH-350	PMX-05R (children) PMXA-OTF20R (adults)	Lixel S-15, Lixel S-25, Lixel S-35
Ligand/carrier	Coating with poly-HEMA	Polymyxin B (covalent bond) polystyrene conjugated fiber	Hexadecyl group; multipore cellulose beads
Mechanism of hemoperfusion	Van der Waals force	Electrostatic interaction; hydrophobic interaction	Hydrophobic interaction; molecular sieving effect
Filling solution	Pyrogen-free sterilized water	Saline (pH 2)	Solution of citric acid and sodium citrate
Amount of adsorbent (g)	100	15/56	150/250/350
Sterilization method	Steam	Steam	Steam
Blood volume for filling (mL)	70	40/135	65/105/177
Housing material	Polypropylene	Polypropylene	Polypropylene or polycarbonate

HEMA poly-hydroxyethylmethacrylate polymer

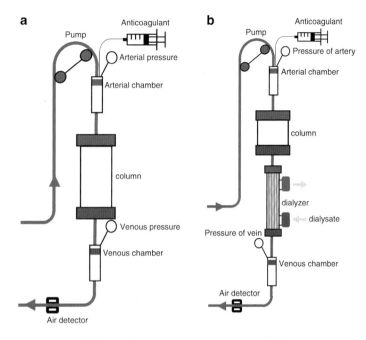

FIGURE 10.1 (a) The hemoperfusion circuit and (b) the circuit of hemoperfusion

The patient should be monitored for reduced platelet levels during and after therapy.

10.2.3   At the End of the Therapy

The column is reversed and set up so the blood flows from the top to the bottom of the circuit.

The blood is collected into a saline or electrolyte solution after the blood flow is decreased to 50 mL/min.

exit

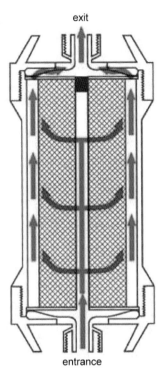

FIGURE 10.2 Blood flow through the column

10.2.4   Maximum Pressure

The pressure to the column should not exceed 500 mmHg.

10.3   Carbon Adsorption

10.3.1   Structure and Principles

Carbon adsorption is nonselective, and therefore, does not require a specific ligand. The process of carbon adsorption of toxic substances is driven by the Van der Waals force. The specific substances that can be adsorbed are determined by the pore diameter and surface area of the carbon column. Covering the carbon with poly-HEMA (poly-hydroxyethyl-methacrylate polymer) decreases production of activated carbon microparticles, clotting, and blood cell damage.

Carbon adsorption has low selectivity for specific substances; however, the adsorption rate for substances weighing 100–5,000 Da is high. Compared with hemodialysis, hemoperfusion is more effective for eliminating substances with a medium molecular weight and those with a high protein-binding rate.

10.3.2   Treatment Parameters

The blood flow rate should be within 100–200 mL/min. The anticoagulant (heparin) dose should be within 1,000–1,500 U/h (initiated at 2,000 U at our hospital). The treatment time should range from 3 to 4 h.

10.3.3   Rinsing and Priming

The saline flow rate should be within 50–100 mL/min (1,000 mL total volume).

More than 500 mL of saline should be used for priming, with a ratio of 5,000 U heparin/1,000 mL saline.

Hypoglycemia can be a problem with hemoperfusion due to glucose adsorption by the column; however, priming with glucose solution is contraindicated because it may induce hemolysis.

10.3.4   Carbon Adsorption

Substances other than the target substance can be adsorbed by a carbon column. Patients should be monitored for hypoglycemia caused by adsorption of glucose. Any glucose supplementation should be injected via a separate line.

Use of nafamostat mesylate, which has a molecular weight of 540 Da, should be avoided.

10.4   Endotoxin Adsorption (PMX-DHP)

10.4.1   Construction and Principles

A column used for the adsorption of endotoxins is constructed of lipid A for endotoxin activation and polymyxin B for endotoxin adsorption. The polymixin B and polystyrene derivative are covalently bonded and formed into a cylindrical adsorbent column of nonwoven fabric. The radial flow design results in a large surface area that prevents pressure loss. The blood should not flow in the wrong direction.

10.4.2   Treatment Parameters

The blood flow rate should be as follows: PMX-05R 20–40 mL/min; PMX-20R 80–120 mL/min.

The dose of anticoagulant should be as follows: Nafamostat mesylate, 30–40 mg/h, heparin 40–60 U/kg initially, followed by 40–60 U/kg/h. Treatment duration is 2 h.

10.4.3   Rinsing and Priming

To stabilize polymyxin B, the packed solution should be acidic, with a pH of 2. Failure to rinse may result in low blood pressure, hemolysis, and shock. Therefore, the PMX-20R should be rinsed with more than 4 L and the PMX-05R with more than 2 L of saline or electrolyte solution.

Saline or 5 % glucose solution with anticoagulant (nafamostat mesylate 20 mg/500 mL or heparin 2,000 U/500 mL) is used for priming.

10.4.4   Therapy for Children

A blood product should be used with a priming volume more than 10 % of circulating blood volume. To avoid hyperkalemia, blood product must be used after hemodialysis or potassium filtration.

Particular attention should be paid to increases in blood volume in children. The treatment should be stopped without retransfusion to avoid volume overload.

10.5   β2 Microglobulin Adsorption

10.5.1   Construction and Principle

A column for adsorption of β2 microglobulin is constructed of a hexadecyl ligand fixed to a porous cellulose carrier. The β2 microglobulin is filtered through the pores of the cellulose beads and adsorbed via hydrophobic bonding with the hexadecyl ligand.

The column usually is placed above the dialyzer when used with hemodialysis.

10.5.2   Target of Treatment

The blood flow volume, dose of anticoagulant, and treatment time should be adjusted according to the hemodialysis parameters used during the procedure.

An S-35 column is commonly used. If the patient's blood pressure drops, an S-25 or S-15 column can be used to decrease the extracorporeal circulating blood volume.

10.5.3   Rinsing and Priming

A solution consisting of citric acid and sodium citrate is used to stabilize the ligands in the column. Failure to rinse may result in hypocalcemia or hypernatremia.

The system should be primed after rinsing to prevent citric acid from flowing into the column. The column should be rinsed first with more than 1,000 mL saline (50–150 mL/min). After the column is rinsedit is connected to the dialyzer and priming is performed with saline and anticoagulant (e.g., heparin 1,000 U/1,000 mL saline).

10.5.4   β2 Microglobulin Adsorption

Substances with a similar molecular weight to b2 microglobulin (4,000–20,000 Da), such as insulin, can also be adsorbed.

Patients can develop anemia as a result of the blood remaining in the column. Increasing the dose of erythropoietin may be alleviate anemia. If anemia remains uncontrolled, a smaller column size should be used or the treatment should be stopped.

Note: Substances Adsorbed with Hemoperfusion

Other intrinsic activated factors in addition to endotoxin can be adsorbed with PMX-DHP. This additional activity became evident due to the effectiveness of PMX-DHP for infection induced by gram-positive bacteria. There is much interest in adsorption of substances such as anandamide, 2-arachidonyl glyceride, and HMGB-1 (high mobility group B-1). Adsorption with PMX-DHP has been reported to be effective for acute lung injury.

With regard to β2 microglobulin adsorption, the effectiveness of adsorption does not parallel β2 microglobulin concentration in the serum. The effectiveness of β2 microglobulin adsorption generally becomes evident within 1 month. As is the case for the PMX-DHP column, the β2 microglobulin column can adsorb other substances, including proinflammatory cytokines.

Chapter 11
Cytapheresis

Yuki Itoh and Maki Tsukamoto

> **Main Points**
> - Cytapheresis is a technique used for removing blood cells from a patient's circulation.
> - Cytapheresis is associated with fewer side effects than other similar treatments.

11.1 Types of Cytapheresis

Cytapheresis is a technique for removing blood cells from a patient's circulation. Granulocytapheresis (GCAP) uses adsorbent beads to remove granulocytes, while leukocytapheresis (LCAP) removes granulocytes, monocytes, and lymphocytes by using a filter. The features of GCAP and LCAP are shown in Table 11.1.

Y. Itoh • M. Tsukamoto (✉)
Department of Nephrology and Endocrinology,
University Hospital, The University of Tokyo, 7-3-1 Hongo,
Bunkyo-ku, Tokyo 113-8655, Japan
e-mail: mtsukamoto-tky@umin.ac.jp

E. Noiri and N. Hanafusa (eds.), *The Concise Manual of Apheresis Therapy,* DOI 10.1007/978-4-431-54412-8_11,
© Springer Japan 2014

TABLE 11.1 Comparison of GCAP and LCAP

Treatment	GCAP	LCAP
Contraindications	Granulocyte <2,000/mm^3 associated with infection	Treatment with angiotensin-converting enzyme inhibitors
Blood volume for treatment	1.5–2.0 L	2.0–4.0 L
Adsorbent	Cellulose acetate	Polyethylene-telephthalate
Adsorption and elimination capacity	Eliminates 30–50 % of granulocytes and monocytes	Eliminates almost 100 % of granulocytes and monocytes and 30–60 % of lymphocytes and platelets

11.2   Efficacy and Side Effects

Cytapheresis is more effective than conventional treatment for rheumatoid arthritis, ulcerative colitis, Crohn's disease, pyoderma gangrenosum, systemic lupus erythematosus, and Behçet disease. Side effects are lower than those associated with conventional therapies such as immunosuppressant drugs.

11.2.1   Efficacy and Side Effects in Ulcerative Colitis

LCAP and GCAP are effective for the treatment of ulcerative colitis. In randomized controlled trials including 120 patients with ulcerative colitis, the efficacy rate was 58.5 % in the group treated with GCAP compared with 44.2 % in the group treated with conventional therapy [1].

An interventional trial in patients with steroid-resistant ulcerative colitis reported 74 % effectiveness in patients treated with LCAP in addition to steroids versus 38 % for patients whose steroid dose was increased [2].

Side effect rates reported in these trials were 8 % in patients treated with GCAP [1] and 24 % in patients treated with LCAP [2]. However, the side effects were not serious. Headache was the most frequently reported side effect.

11.2.2   *Efficacy and Side Effects in Rheumatoid Arthritis*

In a multicenter trial including 38 patients with rheumatoid arthritis who had inadequate responses to disease-modifying antirheumatic drugs (DMARDs), ACR20 (a measure of disease activity and improvement) improved in 69 % of patients treated with cytapheresis [3]. Side effects were transient and not serious.

11.2.3   *Efficacy and Side Effects in Crohn's Disease*

In a clinical trial of 21 patients with Crohn's disease who had active colon lesions resistant to conventional nutrition and medical therapy (Crohn's Disease Activity Index 200–400), the improvement rate with GCAP was 44.4 % and evaluated safety (without side effects) in 90.5 % [4].

11.3   Priming

The extracorporeal circulation system is customized for use with GCAP and LCAP columns. A cassette style circulation system with a monitor for easy priming is used for GCAP. The PlasautoLC system with auto-priming is used for LCAP.

However, extracorporeal systems in use today can be used with low-volume application and can be substituted for either specialized system. The priming method used with a cytapheresis and hemodialysis circuit is illustrated in Fig. 11.1. Priming is the same for GCAP and LCAP, but the rinsing dose differs for each procedure.

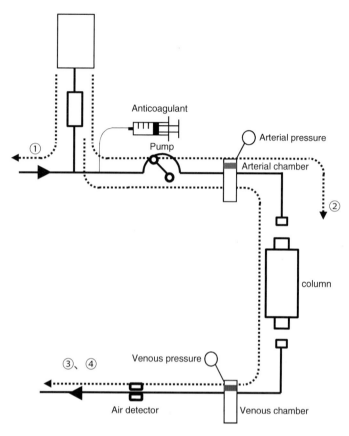

FIGURE 11.1 Priming for cytapheresis: (*1*) set the circuit for blood removal and rinse the blood line to the patient, (*2*) fill the blood removal circuit and connect the column, (*3*) connect and rinse the column and the retransfusion circuit. For GCAP, rinse with at least 1,500 mL with the pump rotating at 100 mL/min. For LCAP, rinse with at least 1,000 mL and (*4*) add 500 mL of anticoagulant solution (e.g., saline with 20 mg nafamostat mesylate)

11.4   Vascular Access

A vein is commonly used for vascular access. However, venous access may be problematic in patients treated with steroids for extended periods or in those suffering from dehydration. In such cases, the central vein can be used for vascular access. In our hospital, removal and retransfusion of blood is performed in each arm separately to avoid recirculation.

11.5   Anticoagulant

The preferred anticoagulant is nafamostat mesylate because patients with indications for cytapheresis often have a high risk for gastrointestinal hemorrhage. Alternative anticoagulants should be used for patients with allergy to nafamostat mesylate. The anticoagulant injection method differs for GCAP and LCAP. In GCAP, nafamostat mesylate is injected at 20–50 mg/h from the anticoagulant line. Heparin is administered at 1,000–3,000 U as one injection at GCAP initiation and maintained at 500–1,500 U/h. In LCAP, 50 mg of nafamostat mesylate in 500 mL of saline is used for the anticoagulant. The nafamostat mesylate solution is injected at 12 % of the blood flow rate and maintained at the same rate throughout therapy. This method of administration is used to avoid blood clotting in the column due to the tendency of the polyester unwoven fabric to induce clotting.

11.6   Points to Note

GCAP is performed for 60 min at the rate of 30 mL/min. LCAP is performed for 60 min with over 2 L of blood at an initial rate of 30 mL/h and maintained at 30–50 mL/h.

Clotting may occur in the column or air trapping chamber. The arterial and venous pressure should be monitored to avoid clotting. Blood removal can be difficult when using a venous access. Avascularization and grasping can solve those problems.

Saline should be infused if hypovolemia occurs. Swinging the column during treatment should be avoided, as it may cause adsorbed blood cells to detach and return to the circulation.

The blood flow rate during reperfusion should be the same as the blood flow rate during treatment. Swinging the column should be avoided during blood removal.

Note: Effectiveness of LCAP for Rheumatoid Arthritis
Rheumatoid arthritis is treated with pulse LCAP using a bigger column (CS-180S) that can process a greater volume of blood (5 L or 100 mL/kg) than the 3 L conventionally treated in patients with ulcerative colitis. Pulse LCAP has been reported to be more effective for treatment of rheumatoid arthritis compared with conventional low volume (3 L) treatment using the CS-100. In some cases, the ACR improved as much as 50–70 % with pulse LCAP [5, 6].

References

1. Shimoyama T et al (1999) Nihon Apheresis Gakkai Zasshi 18:117–131
2. Sawada K et al (2003) Curr Pharm Des 9:307–321
3. Ueki Y et al (2007) Clin Exp Rheumatol 25:810–816
4. Fukuda Y et al (2004) J Gastroenterol 39:1158–1164
5. Onuma S et al (2006) Ther Apher Dial 10:404–411
6. Saito K, Tnaka Y (2009) Nihon Apheresis Gakkai Zasshi 28:218–223

Chapter 12
Cell-Free and Concentrated Ascites Reinfusion Therapy

Norio Hanafusa

Main Points
- Cell-free and concentrated ascites reinfusion therapy (CART) is used for ascites that is refractory to diuretic therapy. CART can increase oncotic pressure and reduce symptoms.
- Serious adverse events are rare, but low-grade body temperature elevation can occur.

12.1 Concepts

Repetitive paracentesis can cause malnutrition that can lead to cachexia from the removal of beneficial substances such as albumin. Ascites can also a impair patient's quality of life by causing an uncomfortable feeling of tension in the abdomen.

N. Hanafusa (✉)
Department of Hemodialysis & Apheresis,
University Hospital, The University of Tokyo, 7-3-1 Hongo,
Bunkyo-ku, Tokyo 113-8655, Japan
e-mail: hanafusa-tky@umin.ac.jp

E. Noiri and N. Hanafusa (eds.), *The Concise Manual*
of Apheresis Therapy, DOI 10.1007/978-4-431-54412-8_12,
© Springer Japan 2014

Cell-free and concentrated ascites reinfusion therapy (CART) is a treatment that removes ascites fluid and processes it to make it suitable for reinfusion while retaining beneficial substances such as albumin. Ordinary therapy for ascites includes sodium restriction or diuretic therapy.

12.2   Scope of Patients

All patients with refractory ascites can be potential candidates for CART, except for the following: (1) those who are suspected of having bacterial peritonitis and whose ascites fluid contains endotoxin, because CART will concentrate existing endotoxin, (2) those who have a circulatory disturbance and may develop hypotension after paracentesis, (3) those who have hemolytic ascites that might cause renal injury, and (4) those who have hyperbilirubinemia (total bilirubin >5 mg/dL) [1].

12.3   Methods

12.3.1   Ascites Fluid Collection

Paracentesis can be performed in an ordinary manner: after an examination of the ascitic area under ultrasonography, paracentesis is performed by puncture through the abdominal wall, avoiding vital organs such as the intestine. The process first begins with local anesthesia delivered into the subcutaneous tissue as well as the peritoneal membrane, then a test puncture is performed using the same needle used for local anesthesia. Afterwards, an 18 gauge needle is used for the puncture to drain the ascites fluid into a designated bag. During paracentesis, the patient's blood pressure or pulse rate and their general status should be closely monitored. Usually, the drainage speed is set to 1–2 L/h and 3 L of fluid

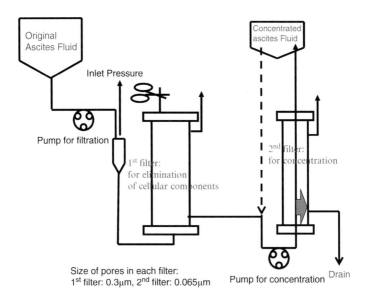

FIGURE 12.1 The CART circuit. The ascites fluid is filtered and concentrated before being reinfused to the patient

in total are usually removed. An electrolyte solution with or without amino acids can be used as a replacement fluid intravenously during paracentesis. If the patient's blood pressure or circulatory status permits, a larger amount of ascites fluid, especially for transudate types, can be removed. However, because removing a large amount of pleural effusion can cause reexpansion pulmonary edema, the amount removed at each drainage session should not exceed 1 L.

12.3.2 Concentration Process

Figure 12.1 illustrates the circuit used for CART ex vivo. This system filtrates and concentrates ascites fluid aseptically.

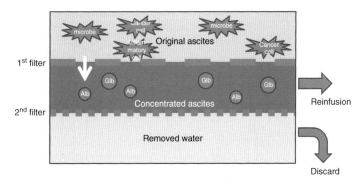

FIGURE 12.2 Conceptual figure of CART. The first filter eliminates cellular components such as cancer cells, inflammatory cells, or microbes. The filtered ascites fluid is further concentrated at the second filter that removes excessive water, and then the concentrated fluid is reinfused

As much as 500 IU/L of heparin can be added to the original ascites fluid to prevent clotting within the circuit, because ascites due to malignancy can contain coagulation factors within the fluid. We almost always use heparin in our facility. The first filter is used to remove cancer cells or microbes within the ascites fluid. This filter is virtually the same as those used in plasma exchange and allows the passage of endotoxin fragments or cytokines.

The second filter is used to remove excessive water and to concentrate the filtered ascites fluid. This filter is virtually the same as those used for hemodialysis. Excess water is removed through ultrafiltration utilizing hydrostatic pressure (differences in height) or resistance (pump and clamp).

Figure 12.2 shows the concepts of filtration and concentration.

12.4   Operation Methods

12.4.1   Filtration and Concentration Process

Processing speed and body temperature elevation are related so slower speeds such as less than 3 L/h or 50 mL/min are appropriate [2]. Filtration from outside of capillaries in the first filter is less likely to raise body temperature [3]; passing ascites fluid from the outside to the inside of the capillaries is considered to reduce shear stress on the cells within the ascites fluid.

12.4.2   Reinfusion Process

A considerable proportion of patients experience body temperature elevation during reinfusion. We usually administer a corticosteroid, such as 100 mg of hydrocorticoid (Hydrocorton™), or we may use nonsteroidal anti-inflammatory drugs. The speed of reinfusion is suggested to be 100–150 mL/h.

12.5   Clinical Benefits

The CART procedure provides benefits due to the removal of ascites fluid and the reinfusion of beneficial proteins such as albumin. We observed marked reduction of symptom scores relating ascites after CART procedure (our unpublished data). Although the clinical benefits of the removal of ascites fluid is not related to the reinfusion process, CART enables the frequent removal of ascites fluid and can improve patient quality of life through the possibility for increased activity and dietary intake, and the reduction of dyspnea. Albumin reinfusion also prevents the hypoalbuminemia that may otherwise result from the removal of the ascites fluid and improves the patient's response to diuretics. In addition, the globulin fraction within the processed ascites fluid can also be reinfused.

12.6   Adverse Events

12.6.1   Body Temperature Elevation

Patients treated with CART sometimes experience elevated body temperature after reinfusion. Cytokines, presumably such as IL-6, are suggested to be the cause [4]. The causes, however, can be multifactorial and have not been exactly determined. Taking preventive measures is important: (1) processing speed should be low (<50 mL/min), (2) the speed of reinfusion should also be low (less than 100–150 mL/min), and (3) medications such as corticosteroids (hydrocortisone 100–200 mg) or acetaminophen can be prescribed before reinfusion. Retrospective analyses at our hospital indicated that a body temperature elevation of 0.4 °C on average was seen among 81 CART procedures [5].

12.6.2   Hypotension

Reinfusion process itself does not directly cause hypotension. Rather, blood pressure decreases may occur during the removal of the ascites fluid. The patient's condition and vital signs should be closely monitored during the entire CART procedure, especially if it is the patient's first such procedure.

12.6.3   Comparison Between Other Therapeutic Options for Refractory Ascites

Other therapeutic options for refractory ascites include the following procedures: (1) paracentesis with albumin infusion, (2) transjugular intrahepatic portosystemic shunt (TIPS), and (3) peritoneovenous shunt (Denver shunt). The advantages and disadvantages are shown in Table 12.1 [5, 6]. Although the CART procedure can cause adverse reactions such as body temperature elevation, the procedure does not have the risk of hepatic encephalopathy as seen with TIPS, nor the risk of congestive heart failure or disseminated intravascular coagulation as seen with peritoneovenous shunt.

Table 12.1 Comparison of therapies for refractory ascites

| Methods | Characteristics | Feasibility | Indication | | Common adverse events |
			Severe jaundice (T-Bil >5 mg/dL)	Poor prognostic patients	
Cell-free and concentrated ascites reinfusion therapy (CART)[a]	Combined removal of ascites fluid and supplementation of proteins. Potential adverse events due to endotoxin reinfusion in patient with liver cirrhosis and bacterial peritonitis	○	×	○	Fever
Paracentesis + albumin infusion	Total albumin replacement for discarded ascites fluid is impossible even with albumin infusion	○	○	○	Progression of hypoalbuminemia and malnutrition circulatory disturbances

(continued)

TABLE 12.1 (continued)

Methods	Characteristics	Feasibility	Indication		Poor prognostic patients	Common adverse events
			Severe jaundice (T-Bil >5 mg/dL)			
Peritoneojugular shunt (P-V shunt)	Ascites fluid is introduced to the jugular vein by a catheter with a check valve. Risk of occlusion and a high rate of complication	×	×		×	DIC, congestive heart failure, sepsis
Transjugular intrahepatic portosystemic shunt (TIPS)	Risks for hepatic encephalopathy, heart failure, pulmonary hypertension, or liver failure	×	×		×	Occlusion of shunt, hepatic encephalopathy

[a]CART has fewer adverse reactions with only a minor elevation of body temperature and has a wider indication than other therapies. *DIC* disseminated intravascular coagulopathy. ○: yes or applicable, ×: no or not applicable.

References

1. Asahi Kasei Medical (2012) Package insert of ascites filter AHF-MO, Tokyo (in Japanese)
2. Takamatsu S et al (2003) The present state of cell-free and concentrated ascites reinfusion therapy (CART) for refractory ascites: focusing on the clinical factors affecting fever as an adverse effect of CART. Kan-Tan-Sui 46(5):663–669 (in Japanese)
3. Japanese CART Study Group, Matsusaki K et al (2011) Novel cell-free and concentrated ascites reinfusion therapy (KM-CART) for refractory ascites associated with cancerous peritonitis: its effect and future perspectives. Int J Clin Oncol 16(4):395–400
4. Nakajima F et al (2001) Relationship between IL-6 levels and fever during ascites reinfusion therapy. Jpn J Soc Dial Ther 34(5):335–338 (in Japanese)
5. Ito T et al (2013) Single center experience of cell-free and concentrated ascites reinfusion therapy in malignancy related ascites. Ther Apher Dial (in press)
6. Japan Society of Hepatology. Management of Decompensated Liver Cirrhosis (2006) Guideline for the treatment of chronic hepatitis 2006. Bunkodo, Tokyo (in Japanese)

Part II
Therapeutic Details

Chapter 13
Choice of Apheresis Therapy

Eisei Noiri

Main Points

- Therapeutic plasma exchange volume is usually 1–1.5 times the patient's plasma volume.
- Selection of a plasma fractionator (second filter) for double filtration plasmapheresis (DFPP) depends on the size of the pathogenic substance.
- Evaluating the adsorption affinity of the pathogen will enhance the efficacy of immunoadsorption therapy.
- A plasma separator (first filter) should not be used for hemodialysis.

E. Noiri (✉)
Department of Hemodialysis & Apheresis, University Hospital,
The University of Tokyo, 7-3-1 Hongo, Bunkyo-ku, Tokyo 113-8655, Japan
e-mail: noiri-tky@umin.ac.jp

E. Noiri and N. Hanafusa (eds.), *The Concise Manual*
of Apheresis Therapy, DOI 10.1007/978-4-431-54412-8_13,
© Springer Japan 2014

131

13.1   Introduction

Almost all physicians' medical actions are, in principle, "additive" therapies conducted by prescription of a drug, whereas apheresis is the opposite, a "subtractive" therapy. The principles of apheresis can be categorized into membrane fractionation, adsorption, and centrifugation. Diffusion, ultrafiltration, and microfiltration are key components of membrane fractionation. The main components of hemodialysis and peritoneal dialysis therapy are diffusion and ultrafiltration. However, microfiltration is the principal process used in apheresis because the goal of apheresis is to prevent the passage of red blood cells (RBCs), white blood cells (WBCs), and other formed elements through the first membrane and allow passage of select plasma proteins through the second membrane.

Adsorption therapy involves two types of therapy: direct adsorption using whole blood, and selective adsorption from plasma after separation by the first membrane. Centrifugation is used to separate cells for blood constituent donation, peripheral blood stem cell donation, and ulcerative colitis therapy. Ex vivo apheresis is applicable to cell-free and concentrated ascites reinfusion therapy (CART) for patients with ascites or pleural effusion from cancer, liver cirrhosis, or other illnesses. This chapter discusses filter selection for treatment of diseases by using microfiltration.

13.2   Way of Thinking of Prescribing Apheresis for Disorders

13.2.1   Simple Plasma Exchange

Plasma exchange (PE) is the fundamental mode of apheresis, and presumably the most prescribed in clinical practice, although disadvantages include the potential for infectious transmission and the need for plasma replacement from healthy volunteers. Irrespective of whether the pathogen is

TABLE 13.1 Filters for simple plasma exchange registered for use in our university hospital

		Plasmaflo™ (Asahi Kasei Medical)		
		OP-02W	OP-05W	OP-08W
Hollow fiber	Material	Polyethylene (coated with ethylene-vinyl alcohol copolymer)		
	Maximum pore size	0.3 μm		
	Membrane surface area	0.2 m²	0.5 m²	0.8 m²
Maximum ultrafiltration pressure for practical use		60 mmHg		
Priming volume	Blood side	25 mL	55 mL	80 mL
	Plasma side	35 mL	75 mL	105 mL
Rough indication by body weight		~25 kg	25–45 kg	45 kg~
Sterilization		γ radiation		

These filters are used as a first membrane (plasma separator) for double filtration plasmapheresis (DFPP)

known or not, PE is the treatment of choice for eliminating putative pathogenic substances in plasma. PE is also used for coagulation factor supplementation. Target diseases include thrombotic thrombocytopenic purpura-hemolytic uremic syndrome (TTP-HUS), fulminant hepatitis, postoperative hepatic failure, ABO incompatible renal transplantation, toxic epidermal necrolysis, systemic lupus erythematosus, and other disorders. When selecting the PE filter, a physician must consider the patient's condition, priming volume, total processed plasma volume, and treatment duration. Table 13.1 presents information for filters registered at our university hospital.

Blood volume is about 7 % of body weight. In patients with anemia, the plasma volume is (1 – Hematocrit) times the blood volume. Therefore, the plasma volume can be calculated by using the following formula.

Plasma volume(L) = (1 – Hematocrit) × 0.07 × Body weight[kg]

The total processed plasma volume ordered should be 1–1.5 times the patient's plasma volume, referred to as 1–1.5 plasma volume.

Plasma exchange sometimes induces hypocalcemia and sodium overload caused by sodium citrate mixed into fresh frozen plasma. An intravenous calcium injection is one solution. Alternatively, hemodialysis in combination with plasma exchange is useful for electrolyte adjustment. For details, please refer to Chap. 4.

13.2.2   Double Filtration Plasmapheresis

After separation of the blood cell components by a first membrane (plasma separator) such as Plasmaflo™, a second filter (plasma fractionator) such as Cascadeflo™ fractionates and removes specific substances having a molecular weight greater than the cut-off level. Therefore, consideration must be given to the molecular weight of the presumptive pathogenic substance or pathogen and to preserving the patient's albumin levels. When the molecular weight of the pathogenic substance or pathogen is sufficiently greater than that of albumin, the substance will be eliminated from plasma without affecting the albumin level. However, when the molecular weight is close to that of albumin, albumin will be lost during treatment, and albumin supplementation will be necessary. Plasma contents that do not pass through the second filter are discarded together with the pathogenic substances. Frequent double filtration plasmapheresis (DFPP) treatments are likely to result in simultaneous loss of immunoglobulin G (IgG) and coagulation factor VIII (factor XIII). Therefore, monitoring and supplementation should be considered. In

TABLE 13.2 Plasma fractionator (second filter) registered for use at our university hospital

		Cascadeflo™ (Asahi Kasei Medical)			
		EC-20W	EC-30W	EC-40W	EC-50W
Hollow fiber	Material	Polyethylene (coated with ethylene-vinyl alcohol copolymer)			
	Average pore size	10 nm	20 nm	30 nm	30 nm
	Membrane surface area	2.0 m²			
Maximum ultrafiltration pressure in practical use		500 mmHg			
Priming volume		150 mL			
Sterilization		γ radiation			

The difference between the EC-40W and the 50W is the number of pores

cryofiltration, the plasma is cooled to 4 °C between the first and second filters to facilitate precipitation for fractionation by the second membrane. Table 13.2 presents information regarding the plasma fractionator (second filter) used at our university hospital. The plasma separator (first filter) is the same as that shown in Table 13.1.

Lipoprotein is targeted for removal in patients with hyperlipidemia. A plasma fractionator (EC-50W) with the largest pore size and number of pores is used because the molecular weight of lipoprotein is 2,400,000 Da, which differs greatly from that of albumin. The chance of losing albumin is negligible and albumin supplementation is unnecessary. When IgG is the target, some albumin will be discarded because the molecular weight of IgG is 200,000–300,000 Da. The EC-20W plasma fractionator is used for this application. The volume of discarded albumin can be estimated before starting DFPP (see Chap. 5) and albumin can be supplemented during the treatment. When IgM, with a molecular weight of 950,000 Da, is the target, the EC-40W fractionator is used.

The total processing volume is determined according to the intravascular or visceral distribution and vascular transmissibility of the target substance. For instance, 1 plasma volume is prescribed for removal of lipoprotein and IgM because these substances are primarily distributed intravascularly. However, 10 % of IgG is distributed in extravascular space, which is about twice the amount distributed intravascularly (see Sect. 13.2.1). Additionally, it is noteworthy that a slight time lag occurs between DFPP and vascular transmission of IgG. Therefore, the total processing volume for IgG removal should be 1.5 times the plasma volume, performed every other day. The level of IgG generally decreases to 50 % after each treatment, depending on the pathologic condition. Three DFPP treatments, performed every other day, will decrease the IgG level to about one-eighth $\left(\frac{1}{2}\right)^3$ of baseline if the IgG production rate is not high. DFPP can effectively decrease IgM in only one treatment because 80 % of IgM is distributed intravascularly. Three consecutive days of treatment will substantially improve the hyperviscosity of myeloma. However, consecutive DFPP treatments are not as effective in reducing IgG levels compared to that for IgM levels, considering the vascular transmission rate and distribution volume. Virus removal and eradication by DFPP (VRAD) with an EC-50W fractionator was recently developed in Japan for elimination of hepatitis C virus (see Chap. 35).

13.2.3   Plasma Adsorption

Plasma adsorption is used to eliminate certain pathogenic substances in the plasma by adsorption after separation by the first filter (plasma separator). After adsorption, all of the plasma is returned to the patient's circulation. Three types of adsorption mechanisms are available in Japan: (1) hydrophobic interaction, (2) electrostatically adsorbed interaction, and (3) ionically bonded interaction. These mechanisms are used to remove substances other than blood cell components.

13.2.3.1 Hydrophobic Adsorption (Used for Myasthenia Gravis, Systemic Lupus Erythematosus, Rheumatoid Arthritis, etc.)

This modality is used for the removal of pathogenic hydrophobic substances. Both the column and pathogen are hydrophobic; thus the pathogenic substance in plasma readily adsorbs to the device. Anti-acetylcholine antibody, anti-muscle specific receptor tyrosine kinase (MuSK) antibody, circulating immune complex, anti-DNA antibody, and rheumatic factor are hydrophobic and can adsorb to a hydrophobic amino-acid device, such as the Immusorba™ PH-350 (phenylalanine) and Immusorba™ TR-350 (tryptophan).

13.2.3.2 Electrostatic Adsorption (Used for Myasthenia Gravis, Systemic Lupus Erythematosus, Antiphospholipid Syndrome, Familial Hyperlipidemia, Arteriosclerosis Obliterans, Focal Glomerular Sclerosis, etc.)

Electrostatic adsorption is removal of a cation-charged substance by electrostatic interaction with an anion-charged device. These devices use dextran sulfate to provide the anionic charge. The device is chosen based on the appropriate pore size for the substance to be eliminated. The Selesorb™ device, having a small pore size, is suitable for adsorption of anti-DNA antibodies and anti-cardiolipin antibodies, whereas the Liposorber™ device, with its larger pore size, is suitable for adsorption of low-density lipoprotein in patients with familial hyperlipidemia, arteriosclerosis obliterans, or focal glomerular sclerosis.

13.2.3.3 Ionically Bonded Adsorption (Used for Hyperbilirubinemia)

Adsorption therapy is considered for patients with an indirect bilirubin level greater than 30 mg/dL to prevent adverse effects of hyperbilirubinemia on the central nervous system. The

Plasorba™ BRS-350 device, made of styrene-di-vinylbenzene copolymer, uses an ionic bonding interaction. When bilirubin binds to the device, an ammonium group is released. Because the biocompatibility of this device is inferior to that of the others, it is primarily used for plasma adsorption.

13.2.4   Blood Adsorption Methods

13.2.4.1   Endotoxin Adsorption

A polymyxin-B-immobilized fiber column (PMX cartridge, Toraymyxin™), developed in Japan in 1994, is an extracorporeal hemoperfusion device that uses polymyxin-B fixed to α-chloroacetamide-methyl polystyrene-derived fibers packed in the cartridge. The prototypical examples of disease-causing endotoxin, lipopolysaccharide (LPS) and lipooligosaccharide (LOS), are found in the outer membranes of various gram-negative bacteria. These bacterial outer membranes consist of the lipid moiety, lipid A and the polysaccharide moiety, 2-keto-3-deoxyoctonate. Lipid A, which is responsible for the toxic effects, has an anion charge because of its phosphate anion. PMX adsorption is accomplished via the following two mechanisms: (1) electrostatic adsorption between lipid A and cationic amino acid in polymyxin-B, and (2) hydrophobic adsorption between the fatty acid moiety in lipid A and the linear structure of methyl octanoic acid in polymyxin-B.

13.2.4.2   Low-Density Lipoprotein (LDL) Adsorption

Apolipoprotein B on the LDL surface has a cationic charge and can bind electrostatically to anionic dextran sulfate (addressed earlier in Sect. 13.2.3.2). This mechanism is used by the Liposorba LA™ for treatment of patients with familial hyperlipidemia and arteriosclerosis obliterans.

13.2.4.3   Chemical Adsorption

Chemical adsorption is accomplished by a hydrophobic interaction with activated charcoal. Micropores of activated charcoal can trap chemical materials reversibly at 500–1,000 kDa. Activated charcoal is not a biocompatible material, but its encapsulation enables adsorption from whole blood without causing platelet activation and hemolysis. The Hemosorba™ CHS-350 device is indicated for treatment of poisoning from sleeping pills, agrichemicals, and anti-arrhythmic drugs.

13.2.4.4 β_2-Amyloid Adsorption

The Lixelle™ device is often prescribed together with hemodialysis for patients with secondary amyloidosis associated with long-term hemodialysis. Hexadecyl-group ligands on porous cellulose beads with a 460 nm pore size are used with this device. The selectivity of adsorption depends on the ligand hydrophobicity and the microporous sieving effect of the bead surface.

13.2.5   Adsorption of White Blood Cell Constituents (Used for Ulcerative Colitis, Crohn Disease, Rheumatoid Arthritis)

Adsorption of specific white blood cell components is effective for the treatment of ulcerative colitis, Crohn disease, and rheumatoid arthritis. The leukocyte apheresis (LCAP) Cellsorba-EX™ device uses non-woven fabric technology to incorporate a polyester ultra-microfiber of 1–3 μm diameter for the removal of monocytes, granulocytes, and lymphoid cells, which have a weak propensity for cell adhesion. Activated platelets also adsorb to this fiber. Filtering by adsorption on the surface of a non-woven fabric can result in clogging by the adsorbed plasma proteins. Although the target processing volume is 2 L, it is important to know that the therapeutic efficacy of a processing volume of 1.5 L is roughly equivalent to that of 2 L.

The Adacolumn™ device, using granulocyte apheresis (GCAP), has bioincompatible cellulose diacetate beads that activate complement 3b (C3b). The activated C3b binds to the surface of the beads and induces C3b-dependent chemotaxis to granulocytes and monocytes, but not to lymphocytes. The efficacy of GCAP has been proven for the treatment of ulcerative colitis and Crohn disease. It is noteworthy that efficacy is not improved by extending the treatment time, which increases the occurrence of side effects. Thus, increasing the treatment time is not recommended.

13.3   Summary

The appearance of the plasma separator (first filter) resembles that of a hemodialysis filter. However, the plasma separator must not be used for hemodialysis because it will engender protein leakage and hemolysis. Physicians in practice should identify and characterize the therapeutic target by using a specific physical finding, certain substance, or biomarkers. Physicians should ensure that the prescribed processing volume for plasma exchange is appropriate for the patient and condition. However, in patients with acute hepatic failure, the combination of a larger plasma exchange processing volume and either hemodiafiltration or continuous hemodiafiltration can curb the development of hepatic encephalopathy. Reducing encephalopathy allows more time for hepatic regeneration and preparation for liver transplantation.

An ongoing clinical study of PMX™ is evaluating the efficacy of the device for inhibiting acute exacerbations of interstitial pneumonia. A clinical study of DFPP in patients with dilated cardiomyopathy, targeting anti-β1 adrenalin receptor antibody, anti-muscarine 2 receptor antibody, and others, is currently ongoing in Japan. These and other developments are expected to broaden the application of these methods in a variety of fields.

Chapter 14
Determination of Dosage and Frequency of Therapy

Norio Hanafusa

Main Points
- An exchange of 1–1.5 times the patient's estimated plasma volume usually results in one-third to one-fourth of the IgG pretreatment concentration just after the session and about one half after reaching equilibrium, because IgG that is distributed outside of the vasculature can migrate from extravascular compartments to inside the blood circulation.
- The distribution volume affects the amount of plasma removed during a single session, while the production rate or diffusion velocity between compartments affects the frequency of treatments.
- Clearance is equal to the exchanged plasma volume in a simple plasma exchange, while clearance is less than the processed volume in double filtration plasmapheresis (DFPP) or plasma adsorption.

N. Hanafusa (✉)
Department of Hemodialysis & Apheresis, University Hospital,
The University of Tokyo, 7-3-1 Hongo, Bunkyo-ku, Tokyo 113-8655, Japan
e-mail: hanafusa-tky@umin.ac.jp

E. Noiri and N. Hanafusa (eds.), *The Concise Manual*
of Apheresis Therapy, DOI 10.1007/978-4-431-54412-8_14,
© Springer Japan 2014

14.1 Introduction

Hemodialysis removes small substances such as uremic toxins and electrolytes. Apheresis has a wider scope in terms of target molecules. The production rate can vary among patients because some patients will have acute illness, while others will have chronic illnesses. Individualized therapy should be considered because the dynamics of target molecules within the circulation in patients with critical illnesses can differ from steady state conditions. Therefore, the dosage or frequency of therapy should be determined according to the dynamics of the targeted pathogenic substance [1, 2]. In this chapter, therapy variables affecting dosage and frequency are discussed.

14.2 IgG Removal

IgG is one of the most important pathogenic substances in autoimmune diseases treated with apheresis. A portion of IgG is distributed outside the vasculature and enters the blood stream slowly compared to the duration of apheresis session. Processing 1–1.5 times the plasma volume decreases IgG concentrations to one-third to one-fourth of the pretreatment level by the end of the session. The amount of IgG outside the vasculature is equal to the amount occurring within the blood vessels. Thus the IgG concentration rises on the day after therapy and finally attains equilibrium at about half the pretreatment value.

Daily treatments might be appropriate for patients with an acute illness requiring rapid removal of pathogenic substances. Efficient IgG removal with limited treatments requires protocols for therapy on alternate or every 2 days, to allow for migration of IgG from outside the vasculature. Plasmapheresis performed every other day efficiently removes the IgG burden within the limitation of reimbursement

Potentially fatal diseases such as alveolar hemorrhage should be treated with daily plasmapheresis together with immunosuppressive therapy to prevent further antibody production [3].

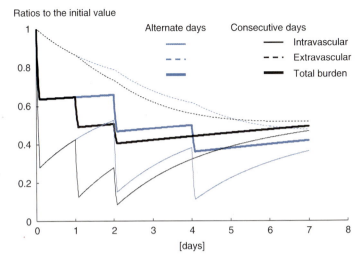

FIGURE 14.1 The effect of treatment schedule on IgG removal. This simulation shows that a rapid decline in intravascular IgG can be achieved with three daily consecutive treatments, while an alternate day regimen of three sessions more effectively decreases both the total IgG burden and intravascular IgG at the end of a 7-day course. Plasmapheresis administered every other day removes more IgG than the same number of treatments administered on consecutive days. Simulation specifications: a 2-compartment model was used. Initial value, 1 mg/dL; body weight, 60 kg; hematocrit, 30 %; processed volume, 1.2 times plasma volume; distribution volume, 0.098 L/kg; 1 % of the difference between the intravascular and extravascular burden moves across the vessel wall per hour

Figure 14.1 shows a simulation of IgG removal with consecutive daily sessions compared with alternate day sessions. The intravascular IgG concentration decreases more rapidly with three consecutive daily treatments, while an alternate day regimen of three sessions more effectively decreases both the total IgG burden and the intravascular IgG by the end of a 7-day course. Therefore, plasmapheresis on an alternate day schedule more effectively removes IgG than the same number of treatments administered on consecutive days.

14.3   Selection of Dosage Prescription

14.3.1   Characteristics of Substances to be Removed

The distribution volume, diffusion velocity between compartments, and production rate of the substance to be removed should be considered when selecting the dosage per session and session frequency. The distribution volume is used to determine the amount of the pathogenic substance remaining after a single session. Diffusion velocity and production rate are used to determine the frequency of therapy sessions.

14.3.1.1   Distribution Volume

The volume of exchanged plasma, processed plasma, and processed blood, which are indicators of dosage in a single session should be determined in the light of distribution volume.

Distribution volume refers to the conceptual volume when a substance would uniformly distribute in the same concentration as in plasma. Distribution volume (V) can be expressed as $V = Q/C$, where Q is the total amount of the substance within the body and C is the concentration of the substance in the plasma. Distribution volume usually is expressed as the volume of the substance per body weight (L/kg). Substances that are distributed only in plasma, blood, the extracellular space, and in the total water content of the body have distribution volumes of 0.05, 0.07, 0.2, and 0.6 L/kg, respectively. Substances with a distribution volume exceeding 0.6 L/kg have good tissue penetration. These substances also penetrate fat tissue, resulting in high concentrations in the fat compartment. Therefore, the apparent volume is large. The concentration at the end of therapy (C_T) is expressed as $C_T = C_0 e^{-KT/V}$, where K, T, V, and C_0 are clearance per unit of time, session duration, distribution volume, and the concentration at the beginning of therapy, respectively, under a single compartment model. Thus, the concentration at the end of the session

TABLE 14.1 Clearance per distribution volume (KT/V) and post/pre ratio (C_T/C_0) and reduction ratio $(1 - C_T/C_0)$

KT/V	C_T/C_0 (Post/pre ratio)	$1 - C_T/C_0$ (Reduction rate)
0.8	0.508	0.492
1.0	0.368	0.632
1.2	0.301	0.699
1.4	0.247	0.753
1.6	0.202	0.798
1.8	0.165	0.835
2.0	0.135	0.865

(C_T) is determined by the ratio of KT (clearance per session) to V (distribution volume). In other words, the concentration at the end of session (C_T) can be estimated by clearance per session normalized by distribution volume.

Table 14.1 shows the relationship between clearance per session normalized by distribution volume (KT/V), the ratios of post- and pre-therapeutic concentrations, and the reduction ratios. For example, a clearance of 1.4 times the distribution volume will reduce the concentration by the end of a session to one-fourth of the concentration at the session start.

Figure 14.2 shows intravascular concentrations and total body burden of a substance at different time points during therapy and the total distribution volume within the body. The decline in the total body burden of a substance is greater for substances with a small distribution volume than for those with a large distribution volume, when treated with the same prescription of clearance.

14.3.1.2 Compartments and Diffusion Velocity Between Compartments

Blood purification therapy removes substances only from plasma. Substances distributed outside of plasma (distribution volume larger than 0.05 L/kg) must enter the blood

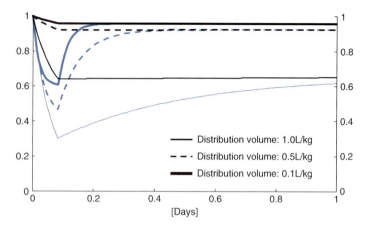

FIGURE 14.2 The effect of distribution volume on removal by plasmapheresis. Substances with a smaller distribution volume are more effectively removed than those with a larger distribution volume when treated with the same prescription. *Pale lines* indicate the intravascular component; *black lines* indicate the total burden within the body. Simulation specifications: a 2-compartment model was used. Initial value, 1 mg/dL; body weight, 60 kg; hematocrit, 30 %; processed volume, 1.2 times plasma volume (clearance, 30 mL/min); and half-life, 21 days; 2 % of the difference between the intravascular and extravascular burden moves across the vessel wall per hour

circulation to be removed. Therefore, the distribution volume outside of the plasma and the velocity at which the substance enters the circulation must be considered.

The body has many compartments containing various substances. The main body compartments are shown in Fig. 14.3. The figure shows how substances move between compartments according to the concentration gradient. These compartments and the velocity at which substances move between them must be taken into account for effective removal of pathogenic substances.

For example, although half of the body's IgG occurs outside of the vasculature, the rate of migration into the

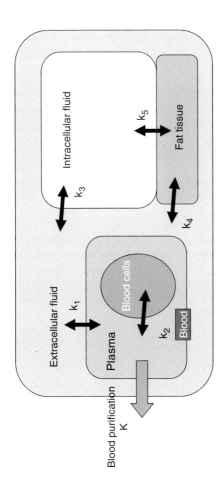

FIGURE 14·3 Compartments within the body. This figure shows the major compartments in the body. Substances move between compartments at various speeds according to the concentration differences within each compartment

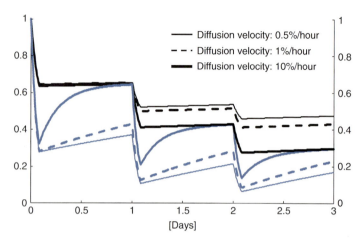

FIGURE 14.4 The effect of diffusion velocity on removal by plasmapheresis. Substances with higher diffusion velocity are effectively removed from the entire body, while substances with slower diffusion are not effectively removed from extravascular compartments. *Pale lines* indicate the course of the intravascular component; *black lines* represent the total burden within the body. Simulation specifications: a 2-compartment model was used. Initial value, 1 mg/dL; body weight, 60 kg; hematocrit, 30 %; processed volume, 1.2 times plasma volume (clearance, 30 mL/min); distribution volume, 0.1 L/kg body weight; half-life, 21 days

circulation is relatively slow (1–2 %/h) [4]. Therefore, during a single therapy session, IgG dynamics follow the single compartment model in which distribution volume is equal to plasma volume. However, after completion of the session, extravascular IgG enters the circulation, resulting in a rebound effect with regard to the plasma concentration.

Figure 14.4 shows the effect of diffusion velocity on the time course of removal. In this example, the distribution volume is set as 0.1 L/kg. Repeat therapies effectively remove substances with a high diffusion velocity, while the same therapies are less effective for removing total burden of substances with a slow velocity.

14.3.1.3   Half-Life and Production Rate

Half-life refers to the time it takes for the concentration of a substance to decrease by one-half due to degradation or elimination. Each substance has a specific half-life [2], although it may be affected by clinical conditions.

The half-life of a substance is closely related to its production rate, making it an important factor in apheresis therapy. Substances with short half-lives, such as cytokines and coagulation factors, have high production rates. Such substances quickly recover their former concentrations, even with frequent apheresis.

In contrast, the production rate generally is slow for substances with longer half-lives, such as IgG and albumin. It takes considerable time for the concentrations of such substances to recover. Thus, repetitive treatments effectively reduce total burden of these substances.

Plasmapheresis performed at the appropriate frequency can be used to reduce the concentration of a pathogenic substance with a slow production rate, such as IgG, while maintaining concentrations of substances with a faster production rate, such as coagulation factors. Albumin has a long half-life and slow production rate, resulting in reduced concentrations with plasmapheresis. Because albumin is critical to maintaining oncotic pressure, it should be supplemented during plasmapheresis.

Figure 14.5 shows the effect of production rate on substance removal by repetitive plasmapheresis therapy. The first session equally reduces the concentrations irrespective of production rates. However, substances with higher production rates recover quickly after the sessions; even repetitive treatments are not effective for reducing their concentrations. The author [1] describes the detailed properties of target substances for apheresis therapy.

14.3.2   Modalities and Their Effects on Clearance

Clearance is almost equal to the exchanged volume in a simple plasma exchange. For example, therapy with an exchange volume of 1.4 times the plasma volume reduces the

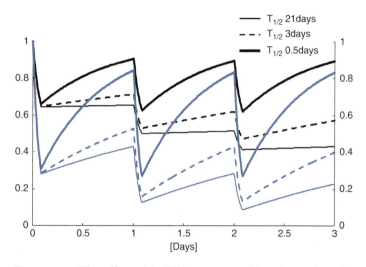

FIGURE 14.5 The effect of half-life on removal by plasmapheresis. Half-life is closely related to production rate. During the first session, the same amount of substance is removed irrespective of half-life. The plasma level and total body burden of a substance with a shorter half-life (i.e., higher production rate) cannot be reduced, even with repeated treatments. *Pale lines* represent the course of the intravascular component and *black lines* the total burden within the body. Simulation specifications: a 2-compartment model was used. Initial value, 1 mg/dL; body weight, 60 kg; hematocrit, 30 %; processed volume, 1.2 times plasma volume (clearance, 30 mL/min); distribution volume, 0.1 L/kg body weight; 1 % of the difference between the intravascular and extravascular burden moves across the vessel wall per hour

concentration of substances limited to the plasma (distribution volume equal to 1 plasma volume) to one-fourth of the initial concentration (Table 14.1).

The second filter used in double filtration plasmapheresis (DFPP) does not fully remove pathogenic substances. For example, a small portion of IgG returns to the circulation. The amount returned depends on the sieving coefficient (SC) of the second filter. An SC of one results in equilibration between the amount removed and the amount returned to circulation. The SC is calculated as the concentration of the filtrate (Cf) divided by the concentration at the filter inlet (Ci) (SC = Cf/Ci).

DFPP clearance corresponds to the processed plasma volume multiplied by 1 minus the SC (1 − SC). For a substance with an SC of 0.3, the processed plasma volume is multiplied by 1 minus 0.3, or 0.7 (processed plasma volume × 0.7 = DFPP clearance). Thus, a processed plasma volume of 1.4 plasma volume results in a DFPP clearance of 37.5 % of the pretreatment value ($e^{-(1.4 \times 0.7)} = 0.375$). The actual SC of the second filter decreases during a session. SC as described here is a conceptual value; it is the ratio of the total amount of substance filtered by the second filter to the total amount that entered the filter during entire session period.

Each type of plasma adsorption column has a maximum adsorption capacity. For example, a tryptophan conjugated column becomes saturated with IgG (excepting subclass IgG4) filtered from up to 2 L of plasma at the usual concentration. Clearance is equal to a processed volume of less than 2 L, while the upper limit of clearance is capped at 2 L. The efficiency of plasma adsorption is lower for patients with a large physique with a larger plasma volume compared to those with a small physique. For example, a processed plasma volume of 2 L in a patient with a weight of 60 kg and 30 % hematocrit (1 PV = 2.9 L) results in reduction to one-half ($e^{-(2/2.9)} = 0.506$) the original concentration. A patient with a body weight of 90 kg and 25 % hematocrit (1 PV = 4.8 L) with the same amount of processed plasma volume will only have a reduction of two-thirds ($e^{-(2/4.8)} = 0.655$) of the beginning concentration. The direct hemoperfusion clearance can be equal to the processed blood volume. The maximum capacity of the column may differ for various substances; this remains to be clarified.

14.3.3   Summary

Distribution volume is a key factor for determining the efficacy of a single apheresis session. The diffusion velocity between compartments and the production rate (half-life) are key factors for determining the frequency of therapy.

Note: Estimation of Plasma Volume

Estimation of the plasma volume is indispensable for determining the appropriate plasmapheresis dosage. As described earlier, the target substance occurs in the plasma. The amount of plasma compared to the estimated total plasma volume determines the course of the concentration during the session.

Blood volume is equal to 7 % of the body weight and plasma corresponds to 1 minus the hematocrit (1 – hematocrit). Therefore, plasma volume is calculated as 0.07 (L/kg) × body weight (kg) × (1 – hematocrit). The value is easily calculated and is used widely in clinical settings. This calculation is used in this text.

Another reported [2] equation for calculating plasma volume is the following: plasma volume (mL) = (1 – hematocrit) × (b + c × body weight [kg]), where b = 1,530 and c = 41.0 for males, and b = 864 and c = 47.2 for females.

References

1. Hanafusa N (2011) Theoretical basis of pathogenic substance removal during plasmapheresis. Ther Apher Dial 15(5):421–430
2. Kaplan AA (2008) Therapeutic plasma exchange: core curriculum 2008. Am J Kidney Dis 52(6):1180–1196
3. Jayne DR et al (2007) Randomized trial of plasma exchange or high-dosage methylprednisolone as adjunctive therapy for severe renal vasculitis. J Am Soc Nephrol 18(7):2180–2188
4. Kaplan AA (1992) Towards a rational prescription of plasma exchange: the kinetics of immunoglobulin removal. Semin Dial 5(3):227–229

Chapter 15
Vascular Access

Koji Okamoto

> **Main Points**
> - Access location and catheter selection
> - Dialysis catheter complications

15.1 Blood Access

When apheresis is chosen, vascular access must be established prior to initiating treatment. The broad categories of vascular access available for apheresis therapy include arteriovenous graft, fistula, direct puncture, and non-tunneled and tunneled catheters, while arteriovenous graft and fistula are generally used for long-term hemodialysis. The choice of modality

K. Okamoto (✉)
Department of Hemodialysis & Apheresis, University Hospital,
The University of Tokyo, 7-3-1 Hongo, Bunkyo-ku, Tokyo 113-8655, Japan
e-mail: okamoto5-tky@umin.ac.jp

E. Noiri and N. Hanafusa (eds.), *The Concise Manual*
of Apheresis Therapy, DOI 10.1007/978-4-431-54412-8_15,
© Springer Japan 2014

depends upon factors such as therapy prevalence and the expected blood flow rate (Q_B), whether the patient will be hospitalized or will be an outpatient, and if there is a preexistent access. Generally, direct puncture or catheter placement is recommended.

15.2   Pre-existing Blood Access During Apheresis

For patients with endstage renal disease (ESRD) undergoing hemodialysis it can be appropriate to use the existing angioaccess (e.g., arteriovenous graft or fistula). In continuous hemodiafiltration (CHDF), continuous hemofiltration (CHF), and plasma exchange (PE) therapy, we recommend catheter-based access because of the blood instability and for easier management of the puncture site. Many events occurring during continuous therapy can jeopardize the existing access.

15.3   Direct Puncture

15.3.1   Direct Artery Puncture

This is a convenient method. However, if the therapy will be administered more than twice a week, other methods are better because of issues with pain, hematoma, and other complications. Care should be taken to avoid damage to the median nerve when using the brachial artery for puncture. It is not suitable for unconscious patients, because of the risk of oversight for nerve damage.

15.3.2   Direct Vein–Vein Puncture

The vein–vein puncture method is used for relatively low Q_B apheresis (not more than 100 mL/min like PE or plasma absorption).

15.3.2.1   Cubital Region

Because the Q_B is not high in the cubital region, recirculation is a problem, and the return route should be placed in another limb. A mild tourniquet cuff can be used to increase the Q_B in the short term, but care should be taken to avoid nerve damage.

15.3.2.2   Femoral Vein

Too much pressure on skin during the puncture of the femoral vein can bend the indwelling needle. It is not a problem if blood overflows without any sign of arterial bleeding. The available Q_B is less than 150 mL/min.

15.4   Blood Access Catheter (Non-tunneled)

There are generally two types of dialysis catheters: tunneled and non-tunneled. A non-tunneled catheter is for short-term use, often for a short-term dialysis session or apheresis. It emerges at the site of entry into the vein. The procedure to insert a non-tunneled catheter takes a maximum of about 60 min.

15.4.1   Locations for Catheter Insertion

15.4.1.1   Internal Jugular Vein

The right internal jugular is the most preferable venous insertion because the left internal jugular may have a low blood flow due to the tight angle to the right heart ventricle. Insertion into the internal jugular vein is associated with a lower risk of infection compared with that into the femoral vein. However, it is difficult to manage and avoid infection in patients with a tracheotomy, because of the short distance from endotracheal tube (Fig. 15.1).

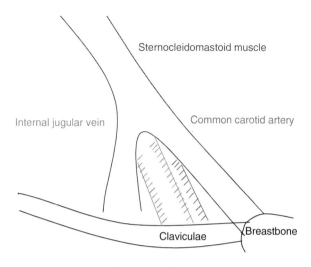

FIGURE 15.1 Anatomy of the insertion area for the right internal jugular vein

15.4.1.2   Femoral Vein

Femoral vein insertion has the biggest risk of infection. The catheter will be moving out and into the insertion site while the patient is sitting and walking, possibly causing a mixing of the heparinized saline and blood that can cause a clot to form. It is best to avoid femoral vein access in patients with high mobility. In the left femoral vein, the tight curve of the aorta near the spinal bone can hamper blood flow (Fig. 15.2).

15.4.1.3   Subclavian Vein

In patients with a high risk of endstage renal disease, insertion into the subclavian vein should be avoided because of the risk of subclavian venous stenosis, which can become a severe problem with blood access on the upper limbs. A catheter inserted in the subclavian vein can be compressed between the clavicle and first rib (pinch-off syndrome). Other risks include uncontrollable hemorrhage, pneumothorax, hemothorax, and subclavian venous occlusion.

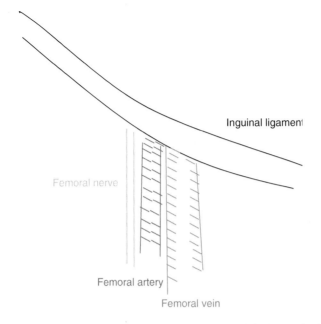

FIGURE 15.2 Anatomy of the insertion area for the right femoral vein

15.4.2   Troubleshooting

15.4.2.1   Complications at the Time of Catheter Insertion

Vascular Injury

Arterial puncture is noted in 3–15 % of central venous access procedures, but immediate recognition and management usually prevents subsequent complications. Once an arterial puncture is suspected, the needle should be immediately withdrawn and direct but nonocclusive pressure applied to the site continuously for 15 min to prevent the formation of hematomas. Unrecognized arterial cannulation with subsequent dilation and catheter placement is associated with life-threatening hemorrhage and neurologic complications. Late recognition of arterial cannulation

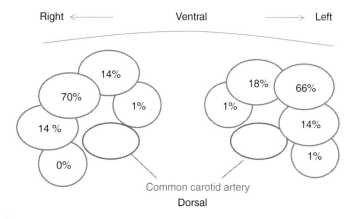

FIGURE 15.3 Anatomical variance of common jugular artery location at the level of annular cartilage [1]

increases the risk of hemorrhagic complications that may require surgical intervention. Procedures should be performed with ultrasound guidance because of the anatomical variance found between patients (Fig. 15.3).

Malposition

The correct placement of the catheter must be confirmed by radiography because clinician judgment does not consistently predict catheter malposition or other mechanical complications, especially for less experienced operators. This is most commonly performed in the operating room and in emergent situations.

Venous Air Embolism

Venipunctures can create a risk for venous air embolism. Air is easily entrained into the vascular space when a needle or catheter is left open to the atmosphere. Fatal doses of air measuring as little as 20 mL can be aspirated in seconds through a large bore catheter. Patients who are in an upright position, hypovolemia state, or spontaneous deep breath during instrumentation as well as practitioner inattention to catheter seals can increase the risk for entraining air. Trendelenburg positioning, the Valsalva maneuver, prompt needle/catheter occlusion, and tight intravenous connections can help to avoid this complication.

15.4.2.2   Complications After Catheter Insertion

Inadequate Blood Flow

Catheters generate negative pressures around their ports as a result of direct fluid extraction and the Bernoulli effect. Catheters are vulnerable to thrombosis, fibrin sheath formation, primary malposition, secondary displacement, or dislocation of the catheter tips. Adherence of the catheter tips to the vein wall can be corrected by reversing catheter ports but this leads to a higher recirculation rate. Other options are to use a guide wire procedure under radiography, or to change the catheter to an end-hole type.

Thrombosis

Both the prevention and treatment of catheter thrombosis are important clinical issues. To prevent thrombus formation, both lumens of the double lumen catheter are instilled with heparin after hemodialysis. The amount injected should only fill the catheter lumen to minimize systemic heparinization, and the length of the catheter determines the appropriate heparin dose. Heparin of either 1 mL = 100 units, 1 mL = 1,000 units, 1 mL = 5,000 units, or 1 mL = 10,000 units can be used. However, the risk of inadvertent anticoagulation has led many centers to abandon the 1:5,000 and 1:10,000 concentrations. Warfarin or low molecular weight heparin may also prevent catheter thrombus due to either intraluminal clot or fibrin sheath formation. Well-controlled trials investigating the effectiveness of partial or systemic anticoagulation are currently underway. The instillation of rtPA, rather than heparin, may improve catheter blood flow and decrease the incidence of catheter clotting. Lytic agents, such as urokinase and rtPA, can be effective as treatment, however, in our experience, many catheters cannot be salvaged with adequate blood flow by the use of thrombolytic agents alone. Non-cuffed catheters should be exchanged if flow is inadequate.

Infection

The following five steps (sometimes called the Pronovost checklist [2] can be followed to reduce catheter-related bloodstream infections: (1) hand hygiene, (2) chlorhexidine skin antisepsis, (3) maximal barrier precautions, (4) avoidance of insertion into the femoral vein, and (5) removal of unnecessary catheters. Additional interventions that may reduce catheter-associated bloodstream infections are as follows: (1) antibiotic impregnated catheters, (2) nursing supervision, and (3) vigilant catheter care.

Note: Catheter Development
In 1969, the use of catheters for hemodialysis was first reported [3]. At that time, two single lumen catheters were placed in the subclavian veins and the contralateral subclavian or femoral vein. In the early 1980s, physicians started to use lumen catheters, which are a hard coaxial type and are replaced after each hemodialysis session. Later, catheters made with a medical silicon gum were developed and are still used today.

References

1. Dickson CS et al (1996) Placement of internal jugular vein central venous catheters: anatomic ultrasound assessment and literature review. Surg Rounds 19:102–107
2. Pronovost P et al (2006) An intervention to decrease catheter-related bloodstream infections in the ICU. N Engl J Med 355: 2725–2732
3. Erben N et al (1969) Experience with routine use of subclavian vein cannulation in hemodialysis. Proc Eur Dial Transplant Assoc 6:59–64

Chapter 16
Anticoagulants

Tetsushi Yamashita and Toshihiro Torato

> **Main Points**
> - Anticoagulants are essential to prevent clotting during apheresis, which uses extracorporeal circuits.
> - When choosing an anticoagulant, one should consider the type of apheresis, the materials used (such as in the adsorption column and filter), and the patient's bleeding risk.
> - Adequate monitoring of clotting function in patients is important for a safe and smooth apheresis procedure.

T. Yamashita (✉)
Department of Nephrology & Endocrinology, School of Medicine,
The University of Tokyo, 7-3-1 Hongo, Bunkyo-ku, Tokyo 113-8655, Japan
e-mail: teyamashita-tky@umin.ac.jp

T. Torato
Department of Hemodialysis & Apheresis, University Hospital,
The University of Tokyo, 7-3-1 Hongo, Bunkyo-ku, Tokyo 113-8655, Japan

E. Noiri and N. Hanafusa (eds.), *The Concise Manual*
of Apheresis Therapy, DOI 10.1007/978-4-431-54412-8_16,
© Springer Japan 2014

16.1   Introduction

Anticoagulants to prevent fibrin thrombus and clotting in the apheresis circuit should be chosen with consideration given to any patient comorbidities and the type of apheresis to be performed. The characteristics, usage, and monitoring of anticoagulants used during apheresis will be reviewed here, in addition to related technical notes.

16.2   Characteristics of Anticoagulants

Clinically we use unfractionated heparin (UFH), low molecular weight heparin (LMWH), nafamostat mesylate (NM), argatroban, or citrate as an anticoagulant during apheresis. The molecular weight, half-life, costs, indications, and technical notes of each anticoagulant are shown in Table 16.1 [1, 2].

16.3   Monitoring Anticoagulant Therapy

Some coagulation tests to monitor anticoagulant efficacy are the activated clotting time (ACT), the factor Xa-activated clotting time (XCT), the activated partial thromboplastin time (APTT), and the Lee-White clotting time test. We usually use the ACT in clinical settings because it takes a short amount of time and does not require the separation of plasma from whole blood. Although the ACT can be performed by the manual addition of an activating agent (e.g., kaolin, celite), automated measuring instruments (e.g., Hemochron®, ACTester®), recently seeing widespread use, can reduce the interobserver variation.

TABLE 16.1 Molecular weight, half-life, costs, indications, and technical notes of each anticoagulant

Anticoagulant	Molecular weight (Da)	Half-life (min)	Costs	Indications	Technical notes
UFH	15,000–18,000 (mean)	45–60	Low	Low bleeding risk	– Exacerbates bleeding – Resistant in patients with a deficiency of antithrombin – Adsorbed with cationic membranes or anion exchange resins – Causes heparin-induced thrombocytopenia – Causes dyslipidemia
LMFH	4,000–6,000	90–120	Moderate	Moderate bleeding risk	– Resistant in patients with a deficiency of antithrombin – Adsorbed with activated charcoal or cationic membranes
NM	540	8	High	Patients with hemorrhagic complications or perioperative Apheresis with cationic membranes or anion exchange resins	– Causes anaphylactic shock – Adsorbed with activated charcoal or anionic membranes

(continued)

TABLE 16.1 (continued)

Anticoagulant	Molecular weight (Da)	Half-life (min)	Costs	Indications	Technical notes
Argatroban	527	30–50	High	Patients with deficiency of antithrombin or patients with HIT	– Exacerbates bleeding – Few diseases covered by insurance
Citrate	192		Low	Apheresis in centrifugal systems or donor apheresis	– Causes hypocalcemia

UFH unfractionated heparin, *LMFH* low molecular weight heparin, *NM* nafamostat mesylate

16.4 How to Use and Choose Anticoagulants

16.4.1 Unfractionated Heparin

UFH was discovered in 1916, and became a common antico-agulant after it was used for human hemodialysis by Haas in 1928 (Haas G. Über Blutauswaschung. Klin Wochenschr. 1928;7:1356–1362). It is extracted from porcine intestinal mucosa or beef lung, and consists of polysaccharides that contain glucosamines and uronic acids. Its molecular weight ranges from 3,000 to 30,000 Da, although its average molecu-lar weight is in the range of 12,000–15,000 Da. It is an indirect thrombin inhibitor that forms complexes with antithrombin, converting this circulating cofactor from a slow to a rapid inactivator of thrombin. Its half-life is 45–60 min. It is the most common anticoagulant used not only during usual apheresis but also during cryofiltration as an adsorbent that uses the characteristics of heparin to form cryogel.

16.4.1.1 Usage and Monitoring

UFH is continuously infused for anticoagulation. The proper dose must be adjusted according to any patient comorbidities and the type of apheresis used because a patient's response to a standard dose varies widely. Generally we adjust the dose to maintain 1.5–2.5 times the baseline clotting time: an ACT of 200–250 s, or an APTT of 50–60 s. We usually administer 1,000–3,000 units of heparin as a bolus at the start of the apheresis, and continuously infuse 1,000–2,000 units per hour afterwards. We are able to monitor the UFH therapy with ACT or APTT testing.

16.4.1.2 Technical Notes

1. UFH exacerbates bleeding in patients with hemorrhagic complications and increases bleeding risk if used in the preoperative period. Although minimum doses of heparin

or regional heparinization with protamine neutralization was used in the past, it is rarely used today because of safety concerns.

2. UFH may induce heparin-induced thrombocytopenia (HIT). If there is a decrease in the patient's platelet count, a thrombosis, or clotting in the circuit, HIT should be suspected and another anticoagulant (e.g., argatroban) should be selected. An assay for heparin-PF4 antibodies also has diagnostic value.

3. Alternative anticoagulants should be used for patients with an inherited or acquired deficiency of antithrombin because this condition causes a resistance to heparin.

4. UFH may elevate triglyceride (TG) and free fatty acid (FFA) levels because it stimulates the release of lipoprotein lipase. It also reduces bone mineral density and activates platelets.

5. Heparin, which is anionic, is adsorbed by cationic membranes or anion exchange resins (bilirubin adsorption).

16.4.2   Low Molecular Weight Heparin

LMWH is an anticoagulant with a molecular weight ranging from 4,000 to 6,000 Da that is obtained by fractionation of polymeric heparin. As with UFH, LMWH inactivates factor Xa, but LMWH has lesser effect on thrombin. While LMWH provides anticoagulation for extracorporeal circuits, it only slightly prolongs the clotting time, and as a result, can be used for patients with a moderate bleeding risk. The characteristics of LMWH are shown in Table 16.2.

16.4.2.1   Usage and Monitoring

LMWH has twice the half-life of UFH, and it is occasionally administered as a single bolus at the start of apheresis. We administer 10 anti-Xa U/kg/h of LMWH as a single dose at the start of the apheresis, or administer 15–20 anti-Xa U/kg of LMWH as a bolus at the start of the apheresis and continuously

TABLE 16.2 Characteristic of LMWH

1. LMWH has a low bleeding risk because of its small effect on thrombin.

2. It can be administered as a single bolus because of its long half-life.

3. It has little effect on lipoprotein lipase.

4. It has little effect on the activation of platelets and on the reduction of bone mineral density.

5. It has a lower incidence of HIT than does UFH.

infuse 7.5–10 anti-Xa U/kg/h afterwards. In both cases, we adjust the doses according to clotting in the apheresis circuit. Monitoring with ACT or APTT testing is not accurate with LMWH because it has little effect on thrombin. Ideally we adjust the dose to maintain an anti-Xa activity of 0.3–0.5 U/mL, but testing for anti-Xa activity takes time. Recently the XCT test was found to correlate with anti-Xa activity [3], and was studied as a monitoring technique for use with LMWH. A test kit for plasma anti-Xa activity (Test Team® heparin S, Sekisui Medical) has been developed.

16.4.2.2   Technical Notes

Because LMWH is adsorbed with activated charcoal, it cannot be used during direct hemoperfusion (DHP) when activated charcoal is used as an adsorbent.

16.4.3   Nafamostat Mesylate

Originally nafamostat mesylate was developed for treatment of acute pancreatitis because it inhibited pancreatic enzymes, but it is used as an anticoagulant during extracorporeal circulation procedures because it also inhibits platelet activation and coagulation enzymes. It is a regional anticoagulant and has little effect on systemic anticoagulation because of its

TABLE 16.3 Characteristic of nafamostat mesylate

1. NM is a regional anticoagulant.

2. It inhibits enzymes from being activated during extracorporeal circulation.

3. It has no effect on lipoprotein lipase.

4. It has no effect on the activation of platelets and on the reduction of bone mineral density.

rapid metabolism and dialyzability. Because of this, it is a first-line anticoagulant for patients who are perioperative or at a high bleeding risk during extracorporeal circulation.

Its molecular weight is about 540 Da and its half-life is about 8 min. It is a serine protease inhibitor that inhibits, among others, thrombin, kallikrein, plasmin, complement, trypsin, and factors XIIa, Xa, and VIIIa. It induces slightly more systemic anticoagulation during apheresis than during hemodialysis because of its dialyzability. It also relieves the anaphylactoid reaction that may happen during LDL apheresis with dextran sulfate columns because it inhibits the kallikrein–kinin system. The characteristics of NM are shown in Table 16.3.

16.4.3.1   Usage and Monitoring

We prime the extracorporeal circuit using normal saline with 20–40 mg NM and then continuously infuse 20–50 mg/h of NM dissolved in a solution of 5 % dextrose in water into the pre-column limb. Although monitoring the procedure with clotting time testing is rare, we can monitor NM therapy with ACT or APTT tests. Celite should be used instead of kaolin as an activating agent when measuring with the ACT test because kaolin adsorbs NM.

16.4.3.2   Technical Notes

1. Because NM is adsorbed with activated charcoal, it cannot be used during apheresis when activated charcoal is used as an adsorbent.

2. It is adsorbed with anionic membranes (e.g., polyacrylo-nitrile) because it is cationic. This is mainly a problem during hemodialysis.
3. It can cause shock or an anaphylactic reaction.
4. It can induce hyperkalemia in patients with reduced renal function.
5. It may be required to re-administer NM into the separated plasma for apheresis systems with a long extracorporeal circuit (e.g., plasma adsorption) because of its short half-life.

16.4.4   Argatroban

Argatroban, with a molecular weight of about 527 Da, is the world's first direct thrombin inhibitor and was developed in Japan. It inhibits thrombin from stimulating fibrin clot formation, platelet activation, and vasoconstriction, and is also effective in patients with HIT. It is neither adsorbed nor dialyzed because it rapidly complexes with thrombin. Its primary indication was limited to patients with an inherited deficiency of antithrombin or those with antithrombin levels of not more than 70 % in situations where heparin was not effective in preventing clotting in the extracorporeal circuit. Later it was approved for preventing thrombosis in patients with type II HIT, and in May 2011 it was approved for anticoagulation during extracorporeal circulation for patients with type II HIT on the condition that use-result surveys of all cases be conducted until sufficient data are collected. This is because there were only a small number of cases in the clinical trial of argatroban in Japan.

16.4.4.1   Usage and Monitoring

We administer 10 mg of argatroban as a bolus at the start of the apheresis and then continuously infuse 25 mg/h. We can monitor the effect of argatroban with ACT or APTT tests because it dose-dependently affects the results. We adjust the dose in the range of 5–40 mg/h according to the presence of clotting in the apheresis circuit.

16.4.4.2   Technical Notes

Argatroban is not appropriate for patients with hemorrhagic complications because it is a strong thrombin inhibitor and its half-life of 30–50 min is relatively long. Dose adjustment is required in the presence of hepatic dysfunction.

16.4.5   Citrate

Citrate chelates calcium and is usually used in centrifugal systems, but it can also be used during other types of apheresis.

16.4.5.1   Usage and Monitoring

Citrate is infused in a fixed ratio to blood flow to maintain the citrate concentration above a certain level in the circuit. We infuse anticoagulant citrate dextrose solution formula A (ACD-A) at a ratio of about 8–10 % of blood flow in centrifugal systems and we monitor the citrate effect with ACT testing in the pre-column limb or by measuring the post-column ionized calcium concentration. We also measure plasma calcium concentration because citrate can induce hypocalcemia.

16.4.5.2   Technical Notes

1. Citrate may cause citrate toxicity that manifests as tetany, hypotension, nausea, vomiting, and dyspnea because it may reduce the concentration of plasma ionized calcium.
2. Citrate toxicity is more likely when fresh frozen plasma (FFP) is used as the replacement fluid for plasma exchange because FFP contains citrate. This should be carefully considered when adjusting the doses (see Chap. 17).
3. Dose adjustment is required in the presence of hepatic dysfunction.
4. Citrate toxicity is more likely with peripheral-blood stem cell collection that takes a long time and needs a high blood flow (see Chap. 35).

5. When hypocalcemia is induced, we infuse calcium preparations, and it is common for us to infuse prophylactic calcium preparations in advance to prevent hypocalcemia.

16.5   Summary

We need to select the proper dose and type of anticoagulant during apheresis according to the patient's comorbidities, possible complications, and concomitant drugs, as well as the type of apheresis used and other considerations. We should also adjust the dose according to the results of ACT testing or the presence of clotting in the apheresis circuit. The standard doses of anticoagulants in our hospital are shown in Table 16.4 [4, 5].

Note: Heparin-Induced Thrombocytopenia

Heparin-induced thrombocytopenia, which is known as a common complication of heparin therapy secondary to bleeding, occurs in the following two types:

Type I: This form is typically characterized by a slight decrease in platelet count that occurs within the first 2 days after heparin initiation and often returns to normal after the reduction or discontinuance of heparin. It is rarely of clinical consequence.

Type II: This form is an immune-mediated disorder characterized by the formation of antibodies against the heparin-platelet factor 4 complex and is associated with a reduction in platelet count greater than 50 % that typically occurs 5–10 days after the initiation of heparin therapy. This disorder frequently causes thrombosis. Occasionally patients have developed this disorder after exposure to only a small amount of heparin because it is an immune-mediated disorder. The most specific diagnostic tests for HIT include heparin-induced platelet aggregation assays, solid phase ELISA immunoassays (recently a diagnostic kit has become commercially available), and others.

Table 16.4 Standard doses of anticoagulants in our hospital

	Doses for continuous infusion		Doses for priming	
	UFH	NM	UFH	NM
Simple plasma exchange Double filtration plasmapheresis	Initial bolus 1,500 U Continuous infusion 1,500 U/h	20–50 mg/h	1,000 U added to 1,000 mL of NS	40 mg of NM dissolved in D5W added to 1,000 mL of NS
Chemical adsorption Hemosorba®	Initial bolus 2,000 U Continuous infusion 2,000–5,000 U/h	No use because of adsorption	5,000 U added to 1,000 mL of NS	No use because of adsorption
Endotoxin adsorption	Initial bolus 40–60 U/kg Continuous infusion 40–60 U/kg/h	30–50 mg/h	2,000 U added to 500 mL of NS	20 mg of NM dissolved in D5W added to 500 mL of NS
Granulocytapheresis	Initial bolus 1,000–3,000 U Continuous infusion 500-1,500 U/h[a]	20–50 mg/h	2,000 U added to 500 mL of NS[a]	20 mg of NM dissolved in D5W added to 500 mL of NS

Leukocytapheresis Cellsorba®	Continuous infusion 1,500–2,500 U/h	50 mg of NM dissolved in D5W added to 500 mL of NS; 12 % of blood flow or 300–800 mL/h	2,000 U added to 500 mL of NS	20 mg of NM dissolved in D5W added to 500 mL of NS
Immunoadsorption Immusorba®	Initial bolus 1,500 U; Continuous infusion 1,000 U/h	20–50 mg/h	1,000 U added to 1,000 mL of NS	40 mg of NM dissolved in D5W added to 1,000 mL of NS
LDL apheresis Liposorba®	Continuous infusion 1,000–1,500 U/h	30–50 mg/h	1,000 U added to 1,000 mL of NS; 500 U added to 500 mL of LR	40 mg of NM added to 500 mL of LR
Bilirubin adsorption Plasorba® Medisorba®	Initial bolus 1,500 U; Continuous infusion 1,500 U/h	20–50 mg/h	1,000 U added to 1,000 mL of NS	40 mg of NM dissolved in D5W added to 1,000 mL of NS 2× set[b]

In all cases, doses should be adjusted according to ACT testing or clotting in the apheresis circuit

UFH unfractionated heparin, LMFH low molecular weight heparin, NM nafamostat mesylate, NS normal saline, D5W 5 % dextrose in water, LR lactated ringer's solution

[a]From the drug information

[b]Relatively large dose because of partial adsorption

References

1. Akizawa T (1996) Kesshojokakizai to kogyokozai no tsukaiwake.
   In: Agishi T (ed) Kesshojokaryoho. Igaku shoin, Tokyo, pp 134–139
2. Amemiya H (2007) Jpn J Apher 26:89–92
3. Kanamori N et al (1990) Yakuri Chiryo 18:2187–2197
4. Kobayashi C (1995) Jpn J Apher 14:474–479
5. Shinoda T (1999) Jpn J Apher 18:136–137

Part III
Complications

Chapter 17
Hypotension

Tsuyoshi Inoue

Main Points
- Hypotension is the most common side effect associated with apheresis therapy, so careful attention to monitor for this condition is needed.
- Hypotension is mainly caused by procedures using extracorporeal circulation, vasovagal reflex, or allergies.
- It is always necessary to predict and prevent the occurrence of hypotension, and to choose medications that will achieve this goal.

T. Inoue (✉)
Division of Nephrology and Endocrinology, School of Medicine,
The University of Tokyo, 7-3-1 Hongo, Bunkyo-ku, Tokyo 113-8655, Japan
e-mail: tsinoue-tky@umin.ac.jp

E. Noiri and N. Hanafusa (eds.), *The Concise Manual*
of Apheresis Therapy, DOI 10.1007/978-4-431-54412-8_17,
© Springer Japan 2014

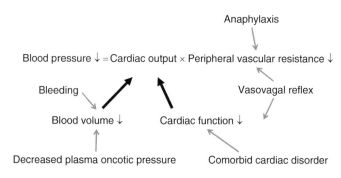

FIGURE 17.1 The main factors of the reduction in blood pressure

17.1   Introduction

A reduction in blood pressure during or immediately after apheresis therapy is the most common side effect for the procedure, and it accounts for approximately 20 % of the reported side effects [1, 2]. In half of the cases reporting this side effect, it is associated with extracorporeal circulation, but some instances are caused by vasovagal reflex or allergy.

17.2   The Cause and Etiology of Hypotension

Apheresis therapy requires extracorporeal circulation and the reduced circulation volume caused by this procedure can lead to hypotension. Blood pressure is regulated by cardiac output (circulation volume and cardiac function) and peripheral vascular resistance, so various factors that are associated with these mechanics can also cause hypotension (Fig. 17.1).

17.2.1   Reduced Cardiac Output

17.2.1.1   Deterioration of Cardiac Function

Critically ill patients often also have reduced cardiac function that can lead to hypotension. Evaluation of cardiac function is suggested prior to apheresis treatment.

17.2.1.2   Decreased Circulation Volume

The removal of a portion of the blood from the body and the addition of saline during extracorporeal circulation procedures can lead to the dilution of blood or decreased plasma oncotic pressure, which can cause a reduction of blood pressure. Compared to that for hemodialysis, the blood volume or plasma volume used in extracorporeal circulation is larger in apheresis treatment, so careful attention is needed when this treatment is initiated.

In addition, plasma oncotic pressure plays an important role in maintaining the concentration of water in the blood vessels, and various factors can lower the oncotic pressure.

Dilution by fresh frozen plasma (FFP): FFP contains a large amount of acid citrate dextrose solution (ACD), which can lead to the dilution of proteins in FFP. The protein concentration in FFP is about 5.0 g/dL, which is quite low compared to that of normal blood plasma. When a large amount of FFP is delivered to the body, a rapid drop of plasma oncotic pressure can occur that will cause a decrease in intravascular volume, subsequently leading to hypotension.

Insufficient replacement volume: When the replacement volume in apheresis treatment is not large enough, oncotic pressure can be decreased. In patients with high levels of serum albumin, or in those with increased serum globulin levels caused by multiple myeloma, replacement using the same volume of 5 % albumin used with plasma exchange might be insufficient. In double filtration plasmapheresis (DFPP), the replacement volume is determined by the patient's serum albumin value and hematocrit value. In either case, blood volume monitoring using devices such as Crit-Line In-Line Monitor™ [In-Line Diagnostics, Kaysville, UT] to observe intradialytic changes in blood volume is suggested. When blood volume is decreased, consider the following procedures: (1) infuse albumin (20 mL/h with 25 % albumin); (2) adjust albumin concentrations; (3) increase the ratio of exchange (the ratio of plasma return/segregation, 1.1); or (4) infuse normal saline (bolus infusion of 100–200 mL normal saline).

Note that it is important to exclude current bleeding in the body as the cause for the blood volume reduction, especially in the patients who have a bleeding tendency.

17.2.2   Reduction in Peripheral Vascular Resistance

To prevent hypotension in cases where it is imminent, the body activates the sympathetic nervous system, which leads to an increase in peripheral vascular resistance. In patients with autonomic neuropathy caused by hypertension and diabetes, such a compensatory reaction does not function properly, and hypotension can occur. In addition, in cases of advanced atherosclerosis, the compliance of blood vessels is reduced, which can easily induce hypotension.

17.2.2.1   Vasovagal Reflex

The pain of blood vessel puncture for apheresis treatment, as well as the anxiety and stress associated with the treatment, can cause a vasovagal reflex.

17.2.2.2   Allergy (See Also Chap. 19; Allergies)

It is necessary to use certain supplies for apheresis treatment, such as anticoagulants and replacement solutions, and allergic reactions can occur to these materials. Attention should be paid to any itching, rashes, or flares of the skin, and edema of the mouth or throat, that occur during the therapy.

Supplies for the Apheresis Treatment

Ethylene oxide gas (EOG), high-pressure steam, and γ-radiation are used for sterilizing the procedure materials. However, EOG sterilized materials can cause an anaphylactoid reaction in some patients.

When absorption columns with a negative charge are used, bradykinin can be induced. Dextran sulfate columns (Liposorber®) for low-density lipoprotein (LDL) absorption therapy and AN-69 membranes used as a dialyzer were the first materials reported as bradykinin inducers. Later, other absorption columns were also revealed to induce bradykinin. Angiotensin-converting enzyme (ACE) inhibitors inhibit the degradation of bradykinin, so when LDL absorption therapy is used in patients taking ACE inhibitors, blood bradykinin levels increase significantly, and this can cause anaphylactic shock. ACE inhibitors are contraindicated for use in apheresis therapy with a bradykinin-inducing material, and so it is necessary to change from ACE inhibitors to ARBs for about 1 month before apheresis.

Anticoagulant

Nafamostat mesylate used as an anticoagulant may prevent bradykinin-related hypotension. However, nafamostat mesylate can induce an allergic reaction, and in some cases anaphylactic shock can develop.

Replacement Solution

There are many reports of allergies to FFP, and therefore careful attention is needed when FFP is used for volume replacement.

17.3   How to Handle Hypotension During Apheresis Treatment

A rapid drop in blood pressure can cause a decrease of blood flow in major organs that can lead to irreversible damage; this necessitates prompt action. One should pay attention to the symptoms relating to hypotension such as yawning, digestive problems, muscle cramps, significant sweating, and a decreased level of consciousness. When hypotension is suspected, the following treatments are immediately needed:

17.3.1   Initial Treatment

- Checking vital signs and the level of consciousness
- Placing the patient in the Trendelenburg position (elevation of the lower extremities)
- Stopping the treatment or drug (when drug allergy is suspected, the blood in the circuit should not be retransfused into the patient)
- Transfusion (bolus administration of 100–200 mL normal saline depending on the situation)
- Supplemental oxygen (as the situation demands)

The initial treatment includes stopping or slowing the rate of ultrafiltration, placing the patient in the Trendelenburg position, decreasing the blood flow rate for the procedure, and restoring intravascular volume.

17.3.2   Treatment According to the Cause

Delay in treatment of hypotension can be fatal, so allergic reactions should always be kept in mind as a possibility. When a drug allergy is suspected, antigen avoidance is critical and retransfusion of the blood in the circuit into the patient should stop. When hypotension is caused by an allergy, 0.3–0.5 mg adrenaline should be immediately administered intramuscularly. See the allergy chapter (Chap. 19) for other treatment methods.

The Trendelenburg position usually improves vasovagal reflex-induced hypotension promptly. In patients with severe hemodynamic instability, atropine sulfate is administered.

Consider the use of a vasopressor prior to the apheresis therapy in patients with decreased cardiac function or a reduction in peripheral vascular resistance (Tables 17.1 and 17.2). In dehydrated patients, a drip infusion should be started before apheresis. Equipment such as Crit-Line In-Line Monitor™ [In-Line Diagnostics, Kaysville, UT] should be used to monitor the change of blood volume when a drop in plasma oncotic pressure is anticipated. Albumin or normal saline should be provided as necessary. In certain patients such as infants with

TABLE 17.1 Oral medicine for hypotension (prescription example)

① Amezinium 10 mg at the initiation or 2 h prior to the end of the treatment

   ➢ Inhibition of norepinephrine reuptake at nerve endings

② Droxidopa 200–400 mg at 60 min prior to the initiation of the treatment

   ➢ Noradrenaline precursor

③ Midodrine 2–4 mg at the initiation or 2 h prior to the end of the treatment

   ➢ α1 agonist

difficulties coping with the decreased circulating volume during extracorporeal circulation, priming the circuit is sometimes done with albumin or red blood cells. Consider dosage reduction on the day of apheresis treatment for patients taking antihypertensive drugs. It is also important to consider and account for diseases that might lower blood pressure such as anemia, hypothyroidism, hypoadrenalism, and sepsis.

17.3.3 Types of Vasopressors and Therapeutic Procedures

The following medications shown in Tables 17.1 and 17.2 are often used in hemodialysis. These medications are also useful for apheresis-related hypotension. The drugs can be administered to patients who have hypotension prior to the treatments.

It is more effective to provide the drug in advance, predicting when hypotension can occur [3].

17.3.4 Therapeutic Protocol

The combination of medications shown in Table 17.2 can be administered to patients who are experiencing hypotension. However, milder treatments for hypotension such as decreasing the priming volume or slowing the rate of ultrafiltration can be useful.

TABLE 17.2 Intravenous or drip infusion drugs for hypotension (prescription example)

I. Maintain plasma osmotic pressure

10–20 mL/h of 25 % albumin (when hypoalbuminemia exists)

II. Maintain extracellular fluid volume

Bolus administration of 100–200 mL normal saline

III. Vasopressor

① Noradrenaline Start at 1 mL/h of 1A (1 mg) in 5 % glucose 20 mL

  ➤ α and β1 agonist

② Dopamine Start at 3 μg/kg per minute

  ➤ Noradrenaline precursor

③ Dobutamine Start at 5 μg/kg per minute

  ➤ β1 agonist

④ Phenylephrine Start at 1 mL/h of 1A (1 mg) in normal saline 10 mL

  ➤ α1 agonist

⑤ Etilefrine Start at 3–4 mL/h of 1A (10 mg) in normal saline 10 mL

  ➤ β agonist and weak α agonist

It is also possible to give phenylephrine and etilefrine as a bolus administration (repeated administrations of 0.1–0.5 mg phenylephrine every 10–15 min, single administration of 2–10 mg etilefrine). In any case, start at a small dose because careful attention to avoid overtreatment is necessary.

17.4   Safety Precautions

It is necessary to choose drugs carefully, and consider the patient's medical situation and contraindications.

References

1. Stegmayr B et al (2008) Transfus Apher Sci 39:247–254
2. Palmer BF, Henrich WL (2008) J Am Soc Nephrol 19:8–11
3. Prakash S et al (2004) Nephrol Dial Transplant 19:2553–2558

Chapter 18
Bleeding Complications and Reduction of Coagulation Factors

Norio Hanafusa

> **Main Points**
> - Bleeding diathesis during apheresis can be caused by anticoagulant drugs, removal of endogenous coagulating factors, or primary diseases.
> - Monitoring is necessary; activated coagulation time as well as direct measurement of fibrinogen and factor XIII levels is indispensable during plasmapheresis with albumin supplementation including double filtration plasmapheresis.

18.1   Introduction

Hemorrhage is an important complication of apheresis. Bleeding diathesis can originate from the use of anticoagulant drugs, the removal of endogenous coagulation factors, or

N. Hanafusa (✉)
Department of Hemodialysis & Apheresis, University Hospital,
The University of Tokyo, 7-3-1 Hongo, Bunkyo-ku, Tokyo 113-8655, Japan
e-mail: hanafusa-tky@umin.ac.jp

E. Noiri and N. Hanafusa (eds.), *The Concise Manual*
of Apheresis Therapy, DOI 10.1007/978-4-431-54412-8_18,
© Springer Japan 2014

187

certain diseases. The complication is well known, but its actual incidence is not high and is reported to be between 0.02 % and 0.2 % [1, 2].

18.2   Use of Anticoagulants

Anticoagulation is indispensable for procedures utilizing extracorporeal blood circulation. The blood flow rate is lower in apheresis procedures than in hemodialysis, and the plasma flow rate in double filtration plasmapheresis or in plasma adsorption is slower still, thus the plasma transit time is long. Subsequently the dosage of anticoagulant drugs tends to be larger than that seen with hemodialysis. Certain diseases also might cause an increased bleeding risk, and in these situations extra care should be taken.

Heparin is usually used for anticoagulation. The ability to remove heparin during plasmapheresis is limited and the half-life of heparin is quite long. Therefore most of the infused heparin enters the systemic circulation. Nafamostat mesylate is often used in Japan as an anticoagulant. The drug works almost exclusively in the hemodialysis circuit because it can be eliminated during dialysis and has a short half-life. However, plasmapheresis removes only a small amount of the drug and it can prolong the coagulation time of systemic blood.

Vascular access site bleeding is sometimes observed during apheresis procedures because a central vein catheter is often inserted just before the session or because native arteries are sometimes used for vascular access. Patients should be carefully monitored during apheresis sessions for bleeding at the puncture site or deep hematomas because anticoagulation agents may promote such complications.

18.3   Removal of Coagulation Factors

Many plasmapheresis modalities, by their nature, are nonspecific in their removal of plasma substances. If such nonspecific therapies do not include supplementation with fresh plasma, levels of coagulation factors are often decreased. For example, plasma exchange with albumin supplementation causes a uniform relative decrease of plasma substances other than albumin.

Double filtration plasmapheresis (DFPP) removes molecules larger than albumin. Figure 18.1 lists the molecular weights and half-lives of coagulation factors [3], as well as of albumin and IgG. Many coagulation factors have a larger molecular weight than albumin and can be removed through DFPP therapy. However, most of them have short half-lives and they recover rapidly before the next session, therefore even with albumin supplementation, the deficiency of such factors may not be obvious.

Fibrinogen and factor XIII (FXIII) have the distinct property of a long half-life, or in other words, a slow production rate, and therefore frequent therapies can decrease levels of these factors [4, 5]. Moreover, reduced production in such cases as liver failure, or increased consumption in such cases as hemorrhage or disseminated intravascular coagulation (DIC), can result in a longer recovery time for such substances by the body.

18.3.1   Importance of Monitoring

Attention should be paid to the reduction of coagulation factors such as fibrinogen or FXIII during plasmapheresis with albumin supplementation. When performing frequent procedures on a patient, physicians should perform direct measurements of fibrinogen and factor XIII as well as coagulation tests such as prothrombin time or activated partial thrombin time.

DFPP is used for the removal of hepatitis C virus (see Chap. 3), and it is recommended that the frequency of therapy be modified according to the fibrinogen concentration. When fibrinogen is decreased to <100 mg/dL, the procedure should be suspended and be postponed until there is recovery of the factor. FXIII does not affect coagulation time

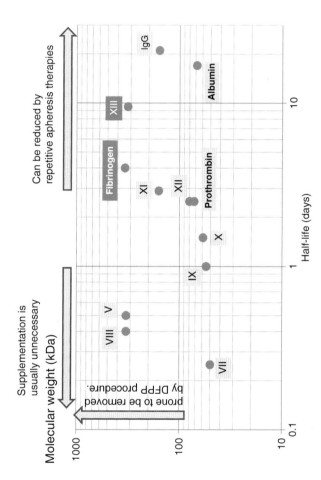

FIGURE 18.1 Half-lives and molecular weights of coagulation factors. Most coagulation factors weigh more than albumin and can be removed through a DFPP procedure. Fibrinogen and FXIII have longer half-lives and can be reduced during frequent apheresis procedures

or bleeding time, but a profound decrease of FXIII is usually observed during frequent apheresis [4]. Therefore direct measurement of the factor is recommended in such circumstances.

The dosage of anticoagulation agents should be carefully modified during the procedures. The removal of coagulation factors results in a decreased requirement for heparin, while the removal of antithrombin III results in an increased requirement for heparin. Activated coagulation time should be monitored for appropriate anticoagulation dosing during procedures.

18.3.2   Measures for Reduced Coagulation Factors

Fibrinogen levels should be maintained at more than 100 mg/dL before the session, while FXIII concentrations should be maintained at more than 5 % after the session. A FXIII level less than 60 % of baseline can be related to an increased incidence of perioperative bleeding complications [6].

The interval between procedures can be increased to wait for recovery of the factors, if possible, when fibrinogen or FXIII levels are reduced. FFP infusion or plasma exchange with FFP supplementation can be considered [7] when the severity of the target disease limits prolonging the interval between procedures.

In chronic conditions where an isolated FXIII reduction is observed, 1 dose (20 mL) of FXIII concentrate (Fibrogammin P) is useful for the recovery of FXIII levels. For example, a patient with a body weight of 60 kg can regain 50 % of FXIII activity after infusion of 1 dose. Patients with a profound decrease of the factor, with levels as low as 10 % before the procedure without a reduction of other factors, may also benefit from FXIII concentrate supplementation [8].

18.4   Bleeding Complications due to Primary Diseases

The target diseases of apheresis include vasculitis (antineu-trophil cytoplasm antibody associated), thrombocytopenic disorders (thrombotic thrombocytopenic purpura, systemic lupus erythematosus, or liver failure), and coagulopathies (liver failure). Hemorrhage or bleeding diathesis can be observed in such conditions.

Nafamostat mesylate should be used and the dosage itself should be made as little as possible. Simple plasma exchange with FFP supplementation should be considered as a thera-peutic modality, because modalities with albumin supplemen-tation can reduce coagulation factors by the end of the session.

FFP or platelet infusion might be considered according to laboratory test results, before placing vascular access, espe-cially for patients requiring central venous access.

Note: Reduction of FXIII Levels During Apheresis Therapies
FXIII makes cross bridges between fibrin molecules and tightens the clot that forms as a result of the coagu-lation cascade. A profound decrease to less than 5 % of normal values often causes fatal bleeding. Even a mod-est decrease causes postoperative bleeding and prolon-gation of wound healing. FXIII is not a member of the coagulation cascade, and does not affect coagulation time or bleeding time. Therefore direct measurement of either the antigen or its activity is necessary to monitor its decrease.

A decrease of FXIII to 10–20% of normal values is often observed during a DFPP course [4]. If major bleeding occurs under such conditions, a further reduc-tion due to bleeding can result in a vicious cycle that can sometimes be fatal [9].

References

1. Mokrzycki MH et al (1994) Therapeutic plasma exchange: complications and management. Am J Kidney Dis 23(6):817–827
2. Kaplan AA (2008) Therapeutic plasma exchange: core curriculum 2008. Am J Kidney Dis 52(6):1180–1196
3. Hanafusa N (2011) Theoretical basis of pathogenic substance removal during plasmapheresis. Ther Apher Dial 15(5):421–430
4. Hanafusa N et al (2007) Double filtration plasmapheresis can decrease factor XIII activity. Ther Apher Dial 11(3):165–170
5. Hanafusa N et al (2010) Virus removal and eradication by modified double filtration plasmapheresis decreases factor XIII levels. Ther Apher Dial 14(3):287–291
6. Gerlach R et al (2000) Factor XIII deficiency and postoperative hemorrhage after neurosurgical procedures. Surg Neurol 54(3):260–264 (discussion 264–265)
7. Hanafusa N et al (2013) The effect of different apheresis modalities on coagulation factor XIII level during antibody removal in ABO-blood type incompatible living related renal transplantation. Transfus Apher Sci (in press)
8. Hanafusa N et al (2010) A patient whose factor XIII level was decreased by double filtrate plasmapheresis and successfully recovered by infusion of factor XIII concentrate. Ther Apher Dial 14(4):432–433
9. Seishima M et al (2009) Decreased factor XIII activity in a patient with subcutaneous bleeding after double filtration plasmapheresis. Ther Apher Dial 13(3):229–231

Chapter 19
Allergies

Motonobu Nakamura

> **Main Points**
> - Some allergic reactions have been reported at the time of apheresis therapy. These complications can be categorized according to the causative therapy or agent.
> - The allergic reaction may progress to anaphylaxis, which may be fatal in severe cases, the immediate intervention is crucial.

M. Nakamura (✉)
Department of Nephrology and Endocrinology,
Graduate School of Medicine, The University of Tokyo,
7-3-1 Hongo, Bunkyo-ku, Tokyo 113-8655, Japan
e-mail: nakamura-stm@umin.ac.jp

E. Noiri and N. Hanafusa (eds.), *The Concise Manual of Apheresis Therapy*, DOI 10.1007/978-4-431-54412-8_19,
© Springer Japan 2014

195

19.1   Introduction

Some allergic reactions have been reported at the time of apheresis therapy. These complications can be categorized according to the causative therapy or agent, as discussed herein.

1. Therapeutic plasma exchange (PEx)
2. Therapeutic sorption (blood adsorption and plasma absorption)
3. Anticoagulant agents

Some studies report few complications with PEx [1–3]. Severe complications and allergic reactions occur less frequently with PEx than with other types of apheresis [4–5].

19.2   Plasma Exchange

19.2.1   Causative Agents

Some proteins contained in fresh frozen plasma can provoke an allergic reaction.

19.2.2   Pathology

Allergic reactions are divided into five types according to their mechanism (Coombs and Gell's classification) [6]. Many allergic reactions that occur with PEx are type 1 allergies caused by IgE. IgE interacts with histamine-producing cells such as mast cells, causing histamine secretion. Histamine secretion may cause vascular dilatation and vascular hyperpermeability. Allergic symptoms begin approximately 10 min after antigen exposure and may include pyrexia, chills, wheezing, or hives. In some patients with allergic symptoms, the allergic reaction may progress to anaphylaxis, which may be fatal in severe cases (3) [7]. Mild allergic reactions may be treated with antihistamine or steroid agents.

19.3   Therapeutic Sorption (Blood Adsorption and Plasma Absorption)

19.3.1   Causative Agents

Allergic reactions caused by anticoagulant agents or angio-tensin-converting enzyme inhibitors (ACEIs) have been reported during therapeutic sorption (blood adsorption and plasma absorption). Symptoms may include flushing, hypotension, pyrexia, chills, wheezing or hives.

19.3.2   Pathology

Immune adsorption devices and dextran sulfuric acid cellulose are negatively charged. Exposure of patient blood to the negatively charged device or cellulose membrane stimulates the metabolic activity of the kallikrein-kinin system, resulting in hyperactivity and increased bradykinin levels. In patients treated with an ACEI who receive apheresis therapy with a negatively charged device or membrane, the ACEI may inhibit bradykinin metabolism, causing bradykinin levels to increase. Increased bradykinin can result in vascular hyper-permeability, leading to allergic symptoms such as facial flushing, hypotension, abdominal pain, etc. Therefore, use of an immune adsorption device or dextran sulfuric acid cellulose is a contraindication for patients treated with ACEIs [8]. In our institution, it is recommended that ACEI be withheld for 1 month prior to apheresis; this recommendation is based on the half-life of ACEIs (Table 19.1).

19.4   Anticoagulant Agents

19.4.1   Causative Agents

Anticoagulants, including heparin and nafamostat mesylate (NM).

TABLE 19.1 The half-life of angiotensin-converting enzyme inhibitors (ACEIs)

ACEI	Half-life (h)
Captopril	2.1
Benazepril	
Imidapril	
Alacepril	7.2
Temocapril	22
Quinapril	23
Lisinopril	34
Cilazapril	53
Perindopril	57
Trandolapril	97–138

19.4.2   Pathology

Allergic reactions to anticoagulant agents have been reported. Most allergic reactions to anticoagulants are type1 reactions. Most allergies to anticoagulants occur with NM. In our institution, a loading dose of NM is not administered for a patient's first treatment because of the higher frequency of anaphylactic reactions with NM compared to that with heparin. NM has a short half-life, which may lead to rapid elevations in blood levels. Although allergic reactions to heparin have also been reported, the frequency is unknown. However, occurrences of heparin-induced thrombocytopenia (HIT) have been widely reported. There are two types of HIT. Although the mechanism of HIT is not known, the onset of type 2 HIT occurs through an immune mechanism. HIT-2 may be severe.

19.5   Treatment for Allergic Reaction

1. In some patients with only minor allergy symptoms, the treatment may continue. However, in principle, in patients with symptoms treatment may have to be discontinued immediately.
2. Patients receiving apheresis therapy are evaluated according to their symptoms.
   - Airway/breathing: hoarseness, a feeling of laryngeal tightness, stridor/wheezing, dyspnea, respiratory arrest, etc.
   - Circulation: hypotension, tachycardia, bradycardia, a feeling of chest tightness, etc.
   - Central nervous system: loss of consciousness, coma, and convulsion
   - Cutaneous symptoms: erythema, reddening, itching, angioedema, and hives
3. The standard treatments for patients with these symptoms in Japan are shown in Table 19.2.

19.6   Prophylaxes of Allergic Reactions

The following steps can be taken to prevent allergic reactions during apheresis therapy. All current patient medications should be reviewed to avoid possible adverse interactions, e.g., check for ACEI use. In patients who show slight symptoms of an allergic reaction before therapy or who have shown mild symptoms after previous therapy, antihistamine agents and steroids can be administered before starting therapy.

Suggested pharmacologic prophylaxes includes the following: an antihistaminic agent (preferably an H1 blocker agent); 25–50 mg of diphenhydramine orally or by intramuscular (IM,) or intravenous (IV) injection; cimetidine 300 mg plus normal saline (NS) 20 mL, IV; corticosteroid; hydrocortisone sodium phosphate 200 mg plus NS 100 mL IV.

Some patients with allergic reactions during PEx may be switched to double filtration plasmapheresis (DFPP) if necessary to remove the causative agents. If a type 1 allergic

TABLE 19.2 Standard treatments in Japan for patients with symptoms of allergy during apheresis

Severe hives

Histamine H1 blocker

Diphenhydramine | 25–50 mg PO, IM, IV | per 2–3 h

Histamine H2 blocker

Cimetidine | 300 mg + normal saline 20 mL IV | per 6–8 h

or

Ranitidine | 50 mg + normal saline 20 mL IV

Allergic bronchospasm or laryngeal edema

Oxygen administration

Inhaled beta agonist | (Ex: salbutamol sulfate 200 mg)

Epinephrine

• Hemodynamically stable patients

0.1–0.2 mg | Subcutaneous injection | Max dose 0.3 mg

• Symptomatic worsening or hemodynamically unstable patients

0.1 mg | Slow IV (2–5 min)

Hypotension

1. Leg elevation

2. Oxygen administration

3. Phenylephrine 0.2–0.5 mg IV (every 10–15 min)

or

Etilefrine hydrochloride 2–5 mg IV

4. If phenylephrine or etilefrine hydrochloride do not improve symptoms, give epinephrine 0.1 mg IV (for 2–5 min)

Bradycardia

1. Leg elevation

2. Oxygen administration

3. Transfusion(extracellular fluid)

4. If transfusion does not improve symptoms, give atropine 0.1–1.0 mg IV

5. If atropine does not improve symptoms, give epinephrine 0.1 mg IV (for 2–5 min)

(continued)

TABLE 19.2   (continued)

Anaphylaxis

1. Call "Code Blue" (emergency situation announced in a hospital or institution in which a patient may need emergent cardiopulmonary stimulation)

2. Oxygen administration

3. If progressing edema of larynx, immediately perform endotracheal intubation or surgical airway control

4. Leg elevation if concurrent with hypotension

5. Stat transfusion therapy (~20 mL/kg): massive transfusion necessary within first 5–10 min

6. Epinephrine 0.1 mg IV

7. Administer H1 blocker (diphenhydramine 25–50 mg)

8. Administer H_2 blocker (Ranitidine 1 mg/kg IV)

9. If bronchospasm continues, administer aminophylline 5 mg/kg IV slowly and inhaled b-agonist

reaction caused by an anticoagulant agent is suspected or if the patient has a history of allergic reaction to anticoagulant agents, the patient should be switched to a different anticoagulant, e.g., a patient allergic to NM may be switched to heparin or argatroban hydrate.

If HIT-2 is suspected or diagnosed, treatment with heparin should be avoided; NM or argatroban hydrate should be used instead. Argatroban hydrate for treatment of HIT-2 should be administered immediately because HIT-2 may cause severe symptoms including arterial and venous thrombosis.

References

1. Goupil R et al (2012) Clin J Am Soc Nephrol 8:416–423
2. Guptill JT et al (2013) Muscle Nerve 47:170–176
3. Kadikoylu G et al (2012) Transfus Apher Sci 47:61–65
4. Basic-Jukic N et al (2005) Ther Apher Dial 5:391–395
5. Bramlage CP et al (2009) J Clin Apher 24(6):225–231
6. Weiss ME, Adkinson NF (1988) Clin Allergy 18:515–540
7. Sutton DM et al (1989) Transfusion 29(2):124–127
8. Owen HG, Brecher ME (1994) Transfusion 34(10):891–894

Chapter 20
Electrolyte Disorders

Motonobu Nakamura

Main Points
- Patients with electrolyte abnormalities, including hypocalcemia, are at risk for developing a life-threatening arrhythmia.
- Many of these electrolyte abnormalities can be prevented with electrocardiographic monitoring and other measures.

M. Nakamura (✉)
Department of Nephrology and Endocrinology, Graduate School
of Medicine, The University of Tokyo, 7-3-1 Hongo, Bunkyo-ku,
Tokyo 113-8655, Japan
e-mail: nakamura-stm@umin.ac.jp

E. Noiri and N. Hanafusa (eds.), *The Concise Manual*
of Apheresis Therapy, DOI 10.1007/978-4-431-54412-8_20,
© Springer Japan 2014

20.1   Introduction

An electrolyte abnormality may occur during apheresis therapy. Electrolyte abnormalities are among the major complications that can occur with plasma exchange (PEx) and double filtration plasmapheresis (DFPP). Electrolyte balance complications reported during apheresis include abnormalities involving calcium, sodium, acid–base balance, potassium, and phosphate levels. Complications with electrolyte balance have been reported in about 2 % of PEx and DFPP procedures, with a rate of about 0–3 % critical or fatal complications [1, 2]. The most common electrolyte abnormality occurring during apheresis is hypocalcemia; Shemin et al. reported a frequency of about 6–8 % [2]. Patients with electrolyte abnormalities, including hypocalcemia, are at risk for developing a life-threatening arrhythmia. Many of these electrolyte abnormalities can be prevented with electrocardiographic monitoring and other measures.

20.2   Calcium

20.2.1   Pathology

Hypocalcemia is the most common complication of electrolyte balance seen in apheresis. Most cases of hypocalcemia are caused by the sodium citrate (acid citrate dextrose [ACD]) in fresh frozen plasma (FFP). ACD chelates calcium in the blood, reducing calcium ionization, which results in hypocalcemia.

20.2.2   Symptoms

Patients with hypocalcemia may experience symptoms of tetany (abnormal sensation around the lips, involuntary muscle contraction, etc.). Furthermore, in advanced hypocalcemia, the plateau phase of cardiac muscle depolarization extends and extension of the QT interval may occur. QT interval extension may result in the onset of a life-threatening arrhythmia.

20.2.3   Prevention and Treatment

In our institution, we administer calcium gluconate at 1 mL per 1 unit of FFP to prevent hypocalcemia. However, we do not use calcium gluconate for patients receiving a combination of apheresis therapy and hemodialysis.

20.3   Sodium

20.3.1   Pathology

Hypernatremia or hyponatremia may occur during apheresis, with hypernatremia being the more common sodium abnormality. Most hypernatremia cases are due to sodium overload caused by the ACD present in FFP.

20.3.2   Symptoms

Most patients with hypernatremia are asymptomatic or have mild muscle cramps, thirst, lethargy. Weakness, illitable and may develop twitching, coma or seizures. However, patients with severe hypernatremia may present with a consciousness disorder, which may be severe or even fatal. Moreover, sodium overload leads to increased extracellular fluid and reduced colloid oncotic pressure, which may result in pulmonary edema.

20.3.3   Prevention and Treatment

The patient's sodium concentration should be monitored every few hours during apheresis therapy. The sodium concentration in patients with chronic kidney disease or endstage renal disease can be controlled with a combination of apheresis therapy and hemodialysis.

20.4   Acid–Base Balance

20.4.1   Pathology

Metabolism of the citrate in ACD results in the production of bicarbonate (HCO_3^-). As a result, patients develop metabolic alkalosis. Patients with liver disease, in particular, should be monitored for metabolic alkalosis because of their reduced capacity to metabolize citrate. Moreover, patients should be monitored for other electrolyte abnormalities because alkalemia may potentially worsen hypocalcemia or hypokalemia.

20.4.2   Symptoms

Patients with mild metabolic alkalosis generally are asymptomatic. However, if the pH rises higher than 7.50, patients may present with muscle fasciculation or tetany.

20.4.3   Prevention and Treatment

Symptomatic patients should be treated immediately. The ACD should be diluted and/or apheresis therapy should be discontinued. Combining apheresis therapy with hemodialysis may prevent the occurrence of metabolic alkalosis.

20.5   Potassium

20.5.1   Pathology

Patients administered replacement fluid consisting of albumin dissolved in saline or other replacement solution may develop hypokalemia due to dilution and removal of potassium. However, hypokalemia may be less frequent with apheresis alone than with combined apheresis therapy and hemodialysis because very little potassium is removed during apheresis therapy alone.

20.5.2   Symptoms

Most patients with mild hypokalemia are asymptomatic. However, moderate or severe hypokalemia (potassium level <2.5 mEq/L) may cause muscle weakness or life-threatening arrhythmia.

20.5.3   Prevention and Treatment

Patients treated with both apheresis therapy and hemodialysis may require potassium replacement or adjustment of the potassium concentration in the dialysis solution.

20.6   Phosphate

20.6.1   Pathology

Hypophosphatemia occurs rarely in patients treated with PEx and blood adsorption therapy. However, patients treated with a combination of apheresis therapy and hemodialysis may develop hypophosphatemia. Patients unable to receive oral nutrition and who do not receive intravenous nutrition are particularly at risk of developing hypophosphatemia.

20.6.2   Symptoms

Although patients with hypophosphatemia generally do not have symptoms, atony of the breathing muscles and an increase in the oxygen affinity of hemoglobin may occur. In such cases, patients experience respiratory arrest or hypoxemia.

20.6.3   Prevention and Treatment

Phosphate levels should be evaluated prior to therapy in patients treated with both apheresis therapy and hemodialysis. Patients who develop hypophosphatemia may need replacement phosphate.

References

1. Basic-Jukic N et al (2005) Ther Apher Dial 5:391–395
2. Shemin D et al (2007) J Clin Apher 22(5):270–276

Chapter 21
Avoiding Complications During Apheresis

Tetsushi Yamashita and Hiroko Yamamoto

> **Main Points**
> - Complications frequently occur during apheresis and should be detected as early as possible.
> - Technicians or operators should fully understand the function and applications of all equipment used and the possible complications of the apheresis procedure.
> - It is important that physicians understand the cause of any complications and manage them quickly.

T. Yamashita (✉)
Department of Nephrology & Endocrinology, School of Medicine,
The University of Tokyo, 7-3-1 Hongo, Bunkyo-ku, Tokyo 113-8655, Japan
e-mail: teyamashita-tky@umin.ac.jp

H. Yamamoto
Department of Hemodialysis & Apheresis, University Hospital,
The University of Tokyo, 7-3-1 Hongo, Bunkyo-ku, Tokyo 113-8655, Japan

E. Noiri and N. Hanafusa (eds.), *The Concise Manual*
of Apheresis Therapy, DOI 10.1007/978-4-431-54412-8_21,
© Springer Japan 2014

21.1   Introduction

Complications frequently occur during apheresis, but they can be prevented from becoming serious if the technicians or operators understand their causes and how to manage them. We will review the complications associated with the apheresis equipment and those associated with the treatment.

21.2   Complications Associated with Apheresis Equipment

21.2.1   Clotting in the Circuit

Blood takes a longer time to pass through the circuit during apheresis than during hemodialysis due to the lower blood flow rate and higher priming volume of the circuit. Therefore, more extensive anticoagulation should be used during apheresis than during hemodialysis. This is especially true during double filtration plasmapheresis (DFPP), where endogenous anticoagulants are removed, and even more anticoagulation is necessary. It is essential that coagulation is monitored by tests such as activated partial thromboplastin time (APTT) or prothrombin time (PT) during apheresis. When pressure in the circuit becomes elevated, even if adequate anticoagulation has been administered, the problem must be quickly remedied because clots can begin to form. The pressure in the circuit needs to be continuously monitored and it is important to prevent loss of blood in the circuit.

21.2.1.1   Cause

Clotting in the circuit can be caused by a deficiency of anticoagulants, formation of white thrombi through platelet activation, frequent blood removal failure, or other reasons.

21.2.1.2   Management

Management of these complications depends on where the clots form in the circuit (Table 21.1) [1].

21.2.2   Equipment Malfunction

Blood purification equipment must have regular maintenance and inspection, as required by the revised Medical Care Act (Act No. 84 of 2006). The operation of these machines should be tested once a month even if they are rarely used.

21.2.2.1   Management

If the therapy cannot continue due to equipment malfunction, we manually return the blood in the circuit to the body with the hand-powered handle, or through other procedures. If there is a spare apparatus, we continue the therapy with a transfer of the circuit.

21.2.3   Human Errors

It is important that operators become skilled in the procedures and use of blood purification equipment. More than one person should monitor all procedures because a delay in the detection of an error could possibly cause serious harm to the patient. In our hospital, we utilize checklists designed according to the type of therapy and machine. They are used after priming, upon starting the machine, before beginning therapy, and before the initiation of plasma separation.

21.2.3.1   Cause

Problems with the procedure can occur due to technician carelessness, insufficient monitoring lack of knowledge, or an

TABLE 21.1 Management according to location of clotting within the circuit

Plasma separator	Elevation of the differential pressure	Search the whole circuit for clots after infusion of about 100 mL of normal saline via the extra infusion line. If there are no clots in the venous drip chamber and the differential pressure (the entrance pressure minus the exit pressure) is over 100 mmHg, exchange the plasma separators[a]
	Elevation of the TMP	If the TMP exceeds the 60 mmHg upper limit of the plasma separators, lower the height of the plasma in the outer layer of the separator, lower the separation rate, and continue the therapy if possible. If the TMP continues to rise over 60 mmHg, cease the therapy or exchange the plasma separators[a]
Blood circuit		Search the whole circuit for clots after infusion of about 100 mL of normal saline via the extra infusion line. If it seems that the therapy cannot achieve the goal, the circuit can be partially or wholly exchanged
Adsorption column		Lower the flow rate along the adsorption column and continue the therapy if possible. Discontinue the therapy if the differential pressure rises over 100 mmHg
Plasma fractionator		Lower the fractionation rate and continue the therapy if possible. If the entrance pressure rises over 350 mmHg, interrupt fractionation and only drain plasma temporarily, or backwash the fractionator
		A device that can monitor the TMP of secondary membranes is available

(continued)

TABLE 21.1 (continued)

Vascular access	Search the whole circuit for clots after infusion of about 100 mL of normal saline via the extra infusion line. If there are no clots in circuit and the venous pressure is elevated, suspect clotting in the access for blood return. If this is present, interrupt the therapy and check whether clots are drawn from the access or whether there is no resistance to saline flushing. Establish a new access if the access is completely occluded. Temporarily return blood to the body via the access for blood removal if establishing another new access will take too much time

TMP transmembrane pressure

[a]There are two ways to exchange plasma separators. One method exchanges only the separators after priming a new separator, the other exchanges all circuits after blood in the circuit is temporarily returned to the body. The safest and most dependable method should be chosen according to technician skill

oversight such as forgetting to lock or unlock Kocher clamp. Problems can also arise from the mistaken entry of air, damage of the circuit, or incorrect setting of the flow rate.

21.2.3.2   Management

The therapy should be interrupted until the patient's safety has been assured. This can involve assessing whether the error has done harm to the patient, sterile conditions have been maintained, and whether an exchange of circuits is necessary, among other considerations. The hospital's risk management plan should be followed.

21.3   Complications Associated with the Apheresis Treatment

Complications affecting the patient's clinical condition should be detected as early as possible thorough monitoring of vital signs and other methods. It is also essential that operators and technicians are trained to manage complications and emergencies that occur during treatment.

21.3.1   Hypotension

Hypotension can occur frequently, and the cause can often be deduced by examining when it occurred. Causes and management of hypotension according to onset time are shown in Table 21.2 [1] (See Chap. 17).

21.3.2   Paresthesias (Citrate Toxicity)

21.3.2.1   Cause

Citrate toxicity results from a temporary reduction in plasma ionized calcium concentration due to exposure to citrate that is contained in anticoagulants used during centrifugal leukocytapheresis or in fresh frozen plasma (FFP) used as replacement fluid in plasma exchange (See 20.2 Calcium).

21.3.2.2   Management

The citrate delivery rate can be lowered (usually along with the blood flow rate) and prophylactic calcium preparations can be infused via the venous return line. The rate of clearance of citrate, which is metabolized by the liver, varies among individuals, and a change of therapy type or combined plasma exchange and dialysis should be considered in patients with both hepatic and renal dysfunction.

TABLE 21.2 Causes and management of hypotension according to onset time

Initial stage of therapy	Cause	This results from a reduction in plasma oncotic pressure due to an infusion of normal saline for priming (initial drop). Careful attention should be paid to hypotension, especially in patients with low body weight or hypoalbuminemia
	Management	Elevate the patient's legs, lower the blood flow rate, interrupt plasma separation, and administer fluids as soon as possible. If pressure recovers, continue the therapy. Lowering the priming volume (no more than 10 % of the patient's intravascular volume) or using 5 % albumin for priming instead, among other procedures, are preventive measures
Thirty minutes after initiation of therapy	Dangerous	An allergic reaction to blood products or drugs, or bradykinin shock
	Management	Cease the therapy as soon as possible. Elevate the patient's legs, return blood to the body if possible, and administer fluids. Changing the drugs used and administering glucocorticoids just before the therapy are preventive measures
	Cause Results from a reduction in plasma oncotic pressure	This results from a removal of a large amount of protein, compared with the volume of replacement with albumin during DFPP
	Management	Adjust the volume of replacement fluid by monitoring the patient's intravascular volume with Crit-Line In-Line Monitor™

(continued)

TABLE 21.2 (continued)

Regardless of the stage of therapy	Cause	This results from vasovagal reflex. It is caused by sympathoinhibition and vagal efferent activation triggered by emotional or orthostatic stress
	Management	Vasovagal reflex, which frequently happens at venipuncture, may happen during therapy. It is important that we relieve the patient's stress. The therapy can usually continue because the condition resolves quickly. Use atropine when there may be serious hemodynamic instability

DFPP double filtration plasmapheresis

TABLE 21.3 Complications during apheresis other than hypotension

Hypertension	Cause	Possibly due to the return of blood, a control of the need to urinate or defecate, or sodium loading by using FFP as the replacement fluid in plasma exchange
	Management	Elevate the head and consider administering antihypertensive drugs if no improvement is seen. In plasma exchange, consider combined hemodialysis
Hematoma/ subcutaneous bleeding	Cause	Due to anticoagulants used during the therapy, antiplatelet agents used as medication on a regular basis, or other causes
	Management	Change or reduce anticoagulants and carefully puncture and stanch the vein
Urination/ defecation	Cause	Possibly caused by extra replacement fluids or hypotension
	Management	Interrupt the therapy if possible. Monitor the patient by assessing vital signs
Palpitation/ headache	Cause	Occurs relatively frequently during leukocytapheresis
	Management	Consider a change of devices

FFP fresh frozen plasma

21.3.3   Other Complications

Other characteristic complications are shown in Table 21.3. We should be familiar with the package inserts of each device used because there are different kinds of complications associated with particular devices.

Reference

1. Iwamoto H (2007) Jpn J Apher 26(1):93–100

Chapter 22
Infections

Osamu Yamazaki

> **Main Points**
> - Early diagnosis, evaluation, and empiric antimicrobial therapy are important for the successful treatment of catheter-related bacteremia.
> - In the setting of a suspected transfusion-transmitted infection from fresh frozen plasma, the transfusion should be stopped and the blood bank should be alerted.
> - It is still unclear whether immunoglobulin complementation therapy is useful for an immunosuppressive state due to plasma exchange.

O. Yamazaki (✉)
Center of Hemodialysis and Apheresis, The University of Tokyo Hospital,
7-3-1 Hongo, Bunkyo-ku, Tokyo 113-0033, Japan
e-mail: osamu195-tky@umin.ac.jp

E. Noiri and N. Hanafusa (eds.), *The Concise Manual
of Apheresis Therapy,* DOI 10.1007/978-4-431-54412-8_22,
© Springer Japan 2014

22.1   Catheter-Related Bacteremia

Central venous catheters were originally introduced as a vascular access for short-term dialysis. At present, double-lumen silastic catheters are the preferred access means for constant use in apheresis. Some groups describe infection rates that are 3.8 % per 1,000 catheter-days in subclavian, 6.1 % in jugular, and 15.7 % in femoral vein catheterization [1]. According to Kidney Disease Outcomes Quality Initiative (KDOQI) guidelines [2], the usage of non-cuffed catheters imparts a greater risk of infection than do cuffed catheters. Regardless, we should carefully evaluate the symptoms of catheter-related infections [3].

The important points of catheter-related bacteremia are as follows:

- Whenever bacteremia is suspected, blood from the catheter tips and at least two blood samples should be cultured.
- Empiric systemic intravenous antimicrobial therapy is administered when dialysis catheter-induced bacteremia is suspected.
- Immediate removal of the infected catheter is generally the best option for achieving a cure of the infection.

22.2   Transfusion-Transmitted Infection with Fresh Frozen Plasma

Transfusion-transmitted infection is an important complication to consider with blood product administration. A single plasma volume exchange with fresh frozen plasma (FFP) represents 10–15 units of FFP from an equal number of donors. Schreiber et al. described that the risks of giving blood during an infectious window period were estimated as follows: for HIV, 1 in 493,000; for HCV, 1 in 103,000; and for HBV, 1 in 63,000 [4]. To minimize the exposure to infectious diseases when plasma is used for replacement, patients should be given large-volume plasma units collected from a single donor rather than multiple single units of FFP.

22.3   Removal of Immunoglobulins due to Plasma Exchange

The removal of immunoglobulins and complement factors during plasma exchange can in theory lead to an immunodeficient state, leaving the patient to prone to infection. It is unclear whether immunoglobulin complementation therapy is useful for an immunosuppressive state due to plasma exchange. In a randomized controlled trial of plasmapheresis in patients with lupus nephritis, patients receiving apheresis were not more prone to infection than other patients receiving a similar immunosuppressive regimen but without plasma exchange [4, 5]. The advantages and disadvantages of FFP and albumin as replacement fluids in plasma exchange are described in Table 22.1.

TABLE 22.1 Characterization of albumin and fresh frozen plasma as replacement fluids in plasma exchange

	Albumin	**Fresh frozen plasma**
Advantages	Low risk of infection and anaphylactic shock	Contains coagulation factors Contains immunoglobulins
Disadvantages	Does not replace coagulation factors Does not replace immunoglobulins	Citrate-induced hypocalcemia High risk of anaphylactic shock

224   O. Yamazaki

References

1. Nagashima G, Kikuchi T, Tsuyuzaki H, Kawano R, Tanaka H, Nemoto H, Taguchi K, Ugajin K (2006) To reduce catheter-related bloodstream infections: is the subclavian route better than the jugular route for central venous catheterization? J Infect Chemother 12:363–365
2. KDOQI (2006) Clinical practice guidelines and clinical practice recommendations 2006 updates hemodialysis adequacy peritoneal dialysis adequacy vascular access. Am J Kidney Dis 48 (Suppl 1):S176–S273
3. Fernández-Cean J, Alvarez A, Burguez S, Baldovinos G, Larre-Borges P, Cha M (2002) Infective endocarditis in chronic haemodialysis: two treatment strategies. Nephrol Dial Transplant 17:2226–2230
4. Schreiber GB, Busch MP, Kleinman SH, Korelitz JJ (1996) The risk of transfusion-transmitted viral infections. The Retrovirus Epidemiology Donor Study. N Engl J Med 334:1685–1690
5. Pohl MA, Lan SP, Berl T (1991) Apheresis does not increase the risk for infection in immunosuppressed patients with severe lupus nephritis. The Lupus Nephritis Collaborative Study Group. Ann Intern Med 114:924–929

Part IV
Autoimmune Disorders

Chapter 23
Neurological Diseases

Masao Iwagami and Kousuke Negishi

Main Points

General Principles

- The effect of apheresis on several neurological disorders has been evaluated in studies with high-level evidence such as randomized controlled trials.
- Immunoadsorption plasmapheresis (IAPP) is generally recommended for neurological disorders, while double filtration plasmapheresis (DFPP) or plasma exchange (PE) should be considered for non-responders to IAPP.

M. Iwagami (✉)
Department of Hemodialysis & Apheresis, University Hospital,
The University of Tokyo, 7-3-1 Hongo, Bunkyo-ku, Tokyo 113-8655, Japan
e-mail: iwagami-tky@umin.ac.jp

K. Negishi
Department of Internal Medicine, Nephrology, Toshiba General Hospital,
6-3-22 Higashi-Ohi, Shinagawa-ku, Tokyo 140-8522, Japan
e-mail: knegishi-tky@umin.ac.jp

E. Noiri and N. Hanafusa (eds.), *The Concise Manual*
of Apheresis Therapy, DOI 10.1007/978-4-431-54412-8_23,
© Springer Japan 2014

Myasthenia Gravis

- IAPP is recommended for antiacetylcholine receptor antibody (A6chR)-positive myasthenia gravis (MG) and DFPP is for muscle-specific tyrosine kinase (MuSK)-positive MG.

Lambert–Eaton Myasthenic Syndrome

- PE is generally recommended for Lambert–Eaton myasthenic syndrome, although it takes a long time to see improvement.

Guillain–Barre Syndrome

- The effect of apheresis on severe or rapidly progressive Guillain–Barre syndrome has been established and IAPP is generally recommended.

Chronic Inflammatory Demyelinating Polyradiculoneuropathy

- IAPP is effective for relapsing-remitting chronic inflammatory demyelinating polyradiculoneuropathy.

Multiple Sclerosis

- IAPP is effective for remitting-relapsing multiple sclerosis (MS), while apheresis may not be as efficacious for chronic progressive MS.

23.1   General Principles

23.1.1   Evidence Concerning Disorders Indicated for Apheresis

For myasthenia gravis (MG) in which causative autoantibodies are identified, and polyneuropathy- monoclonal gammopathy of undetermined significance (MGUS) with an abnormally high level of monoclonal immunoglobulin, apheresis is a sensible treatment modality because it reliably removes these

TABLE 23.1 Usefulness and evidence level of apheresis for neurological disorders

	Diseases	Evidence level[a]
Highly recommendable (level A)	GBS	Class I
	CIDP	Class I
	Polyneuropathy-MGUS (IgG, IgA)	Class I
	MG	Class III
Recommendable (level B)	MS	Class I/II
	LEMS	Class II
	Cryoglobulinemic polyneuropathy	Class II
Undetermined (level C)	Polyneuropathy-MGUS (IgM)	Class I

Adapted from [1, 2]
[a]Class I: Evidence provided by one or more well designed randomized controlled clinical trials. Class II: Evidence provided by one or more well designed clinical studies such as case control studies and cohort studies. Class III: Evidence provided by expert opinion, nonrandomized historical controls or case reports of one or more. *GBS* Guillain–Barre syndrome, *CIDP* chronic inflammatory demyelinating polyradiculoneuropathy, *Polyneuropathy-MGUS* polyneuropathy with monoclonal gammopathy of undetermined significance, *MG* myasthenia gravis, *MS* multiple sclerosis, *LEMS* Lambert–Eaton myasthenic syndrome

substances. However, in many other neurological disorders, the causative substances or mechanisms have yet to be determined. Therefore, it was agreed at the NIH Consensus Conference in 1986 that apheresis for these diseases should be limited to cases where severe neurological disturbance persists without improvement.

Apheresis has been shown to be useful in treating some neurological conditions (Table 23.1) [1, 2]. While the evidence level of apheresis for MG is class III, the pathological roles of MG autoantibodies have been elucidated and the effectiveness of apheresis in removing these autoantibodies has been well recognized. However, randomized controlled trials (RCTs) are needed to produce class I evidence that support the utility of apheresis for MG.

The efficacy of apheresis has been reported in several other neurological disorders that are not listed in Table 23.1 because of a low-level of evidence (below class III). These include stiff-person syndrome, Isaac's syndrome, Refsum's disease, Rasmussen's encephalitis, paraneoplastic cerebellar degeneration, HTLV-1-associated myelopathy, and acute disseminated encephalomyelitis. High-level evidence studies, including RCTs, are difficult to carry out for these severe and rare diseases.

23.1.2   Methods

23.1.2.1   Limited Reimbursement Under the Japanese Health Insurance System

Costs of treating MG, Guillain–Barre syndrome (GBS), chronic inflammatory demyelinating polyradiculoneuropathy (CIDP), and multiple sclerosis (MS) are reimbursed for up to 7 sessions per month and for up to 3 months.

23.1.2.2   Modality

There have been more reports on immunoadsorption plasmapheresis (IAPP) and double filtration plasmapheresis (DFPP) in Japan, whereas plasma exchange (PE) has been more popular in Europe and America. IAPP, which does not require replacement solutions, is generally recommended for safety reasons, except for special pathological conditions. However, when there is no response to IAPP, then DFPP or PE should be considered. The target volume of plasma treated is 2–2.5 L regardless of body weight for IAPP and 1–1.5 plasma volumes (PV) for DFPP and PE. PV (in liters) is calculated as $0.07 \times$ body weight $[kg] \times (1-0.01 \times$ hematocrit $[\%])$. Heparin is usually recommended as an anticoagulant, whereas nafamostat mesylate is preferred for patients with bleeding tendencies.

23.1.3 Points to Note

23.1.3.1 Allergic Reactions

When blood is in contact with artificial materials in the extracorporeal circuit such as adsorbents, membrane filters, blood circuits, indwelling catheters, and anticoagulants, there is a risk of developing allergic reactions that can cause the following effects: hypotension, shock, anaphylaxis, headache, nausea, vomiting, arrhythmia, dyspnea, thrombosis, bleeding tendency caused by reduced platelets or fibrinogen, or others. Therefore, vital signs should be monitored routinely, and electrocardiographic monitoring should be performed as needed.

23.1.3.2 Adsorption–Desorption Phenomenon

In IAPP, adsorbed substances such as immunoglobulins, complement components, and cytokines may be desorbed. In particular, desorption of bradykinin or C5a can lead to hypotension and shock, and patients should be carefully monitored for these conditions.

23.1.3.3 Infection

Implementation of appropriate infection control measures, such as keeping the catheter insertion point clean and changing catheters regularly, is essential when the catheter is left in place for an extended period of time, because many patients are in poor general condition or are in a severely immuno-suppressed state.

23.1.3.4   Hemodynamic Changes

Careful monitoring of hemodynamics is important because hypotension resulting from an autonomic disturbance might occur during apheresis, particularly in patients with neurological disorders.

23.2   Myasthenia Gravis (MG)

23.2.1   Targeted Substances and Disease Characteristics

23.2.1.1   Targeted Substances

- Anti-acetylcholine receptor (AchR) antibody (IgG1 and IgG3 subclasses predominant)
- Anti-muscle specific tyrosine kinase (MuSK) antibody (IgG4 subclass predominant)

23.2.1.2   Disease Characteristics

MG is an autoimmune disease in which impairment of neuromuscular transmission is caused mostly by antibodies against AchR in the postsynaptic membrane of the neuromuscular junction. Anti-AchR antibodies are present in approximately 80 % of patients with MG, although the severity of the disease is not correlated with the plasma concentration of the antibodies. Anti-MuSK antibodies have been found in some patients without detectable anti-AchR antibodies, suggesting that dysfunction of MuSK may affect neuromuscular transmission. Patients who are seronegative for both AChR and MuSK are classified as having double-seronegative MG, though the presence of other antibodies has been suggested, such as autoantibodies to lipoprotein-related protein 4 (LRP4), ryanodine receptor, and titin.

The clinical features of MG include predominantly proximal skeletal muscle weakness and easy muscle fatigue, which are induced by exercise and improved by rest, in addition to symptoms such as diplopia, ptosis, dysphagia, dysarthria, respiratory insufficiency, and a diurnal variation of symptoms. MG is twice as common in women as in men, and occurs frequently in children under the age of 10 years, women between 20–40 years of age, and men aged between 40–50 years. MG is associated with thymic hyperplasia (60–70 %), thymoma (10–20 %), hyperthyroidism, systemic lupus erythematosus, and rheumatoid arthritis.

23.2.1.3   Treatment

In MG cases complicated with thymoma, thymectomy should be performed at the early stages of the disease process. Anticholinesterase agents are the standard first-line treatment for MG, and glucocorticoids and immunosuppressants are used for long-term control of the symptoms of the disease. Apheresis is considered for life-threatening conditions called "myasthenic crisis", refractory cases with systemic involvement, patients that do not tolerate glucocorticoids or immunosuppressants, and for prethymectomy preparation. Improvement of clinical symptoms is often observed by the end of the third session.

In addition, it has been reported that intravenous immunoglobulin (IVIG) was effective for moderate to severe MG in both anti-AchR-positive and anti-MuSK-positive cases in a RCT [3]. There have been several studies comparing apheresis and IVIG. While a RCT revealed that IVIG had similar efficacy as did apheresis [4], recently published research from Shanghai has shown that DFPP or IAPP improved late-onset MG more rapidly and effectively than did IVIG [5]. In Japan, a RCT comparing apheresis and IVIG is now in progress.

23.2.2   Methods

23.2.2.1   Limited Reimbursement Under the Japanese Health Insurance System

The cost of treatment for MG is reimbursed for up to 7 sessions per month and for up to 3 months under the Japanese health insurance system.

23.2.2.2   Modality

For anti-AchR-positive MG, IAPP has been reported to be as effective as PE and DFPP [6, 7]. Therefore, IAPP, which does not require any replacement solution, is highly recommended in terms of safety and convenience. Immusorba TR-350® containing tryptophan as a ligand is commonly used, because tryptophan has a high affinity for anti-AchR antibodies through hydrophobic interactions. For anti-MuSK-positive MG, PE or DFPP is recommended, because a Japanese study showed that the affinity of the adsorption column of IAPP is IgG subclass-dependent and that the affinity for anti-MuSK antibodies (IgG4) is much lower than that for anti-AchR antibodies (IgG1·IgG3), often resulting in desorption.

23.2.2.3   Treatment Schedule

A typical treatment schedule starts with a total of 5–6 sessions on consecutive days or every other day over a period of 10–14 days, and then once every 2–3 weeks until improvement of symptoms. When a dose reduction of glucocorticoids and immunosuppressants is required, an additional apheresis treatment once every 2–3 weeks should be considered.

23.3   Lambert–Eaton Myasthenic Syndrome

23.3.1   Targeted Substances and Disease Characteristics

23.3.1.1   Targeted Substances

- Autoantibodies to voltage-gated calcium channels (VGCC)

23.3.1.2   Disease Characteristics

LEMS presents as muscle weakness due to reduced acetylcholine release from presynaptic nerve terminals. The acetylcholine release requires an influx of calcium, and autoantibodies to VGCC hamper this release in neuromuscular junctions. LEMS is often complicated with malignancies such as small cell lung cancer, a condition known as paraneoplastic syndrome. LEMS is also common in middle and older aged men, and patients manifest proximal dominant muscle weakness of the lower limbs, an increased thirst, and autonomic symptoms such as impotence. Nerve conduction studies are useful for diagnosis.

23.3.1.3   Treatment

When malignancy is detected, treatment of the neoplasm should be prioritized, which may lead to improvement of LEMS. PE in combination with glucocorticoids or immunosuppressants have been shown to be effective [8]. Apheresis may be considered for patients with a suboptimal response to acetylcholinesterase inhibitors, glucocorticoids, immunosuppressive agents, or drugs that enhance acetylcholine release.

23.3.2   Methods

23.3.2.1   Limited Reimbursement Under the Japanese Health Insurance System

For the time being, the cost of apheresis for LEMS is not reimbursed under the Japanese health insurance system.

23.3.2.2   Modality

PE has been the focus of research in LEMS so far, and there are few studies comparing PE and DFPP or IAPP.

23.3.2.3   Treatment Schedule

A treatment schedule similar to that for MG is recommended (see Sect. 23.2.2.3), but it usually takes longer to see an improvement of the symptoms of LEMS.

Note: Apheresis for Isaac's Syndrome
Isaac's syndrome is a disease in which autoantibodies to voltage-gated potassium channels (VGKC) cause systemic muscle spasm and stiffness. Research has shown that apheresis is effective in removing the antibodies [9].

> **Note: Apheresis for N-Methyl-D-Aspartate Receptor (NMDAR) Encephalitis**
> NMDAR encephalitis is paraneoplastic encephalitis typically accompanied by ovarian teratoma, though there are also cases without tumors. Symptoms of MNDAR include psychiatric manifestations, confusion, memory disturbance, involuntary movement, and convulsion, which may improve with resection of the ovarian teratoma. In a small study, PE was used in addition to immunosuppressive therapy and was found to be effective when started in the early course of NMDAR encephalitis [10].

23.4 Guillain–Barre Syndrome

23.4.1 Targeted Substances and Disease Characteristics

23.4.1.1 Targeted Substances

Axonal type GBS: Autoantibodies to ganglioside GM1, GD1a, etc. (IgG, IgM, IgA)

Demyelinating type GBS: Autoantibodies have not yet been identified.

Besides the removal of autoantibodies, apheresis is thought to show efficacy through the removal of immune complex, complement components, and inflammatory cytokines including TNF-α, IFN-γ, and IL-2, and to cause a suppression of activated T cells.

23.4.1.2 Disease Characteristics

GBS is a polyneuropathy that manifests as flaccid paralysis of the limbs and a disappearance of deep reflexes. It is triggered by bacterial or viral infection (most commonly by *Campylobacter jejuni*). GBS is classified into two types; demyelinating type GBS in which injury starts from the myelin sheath of peripheral nerves, and axonal type GBS that starts with axonal injury and shows delayed recovery. *Campylobacter* infection often leads to axonal type GBS.

Laboratory features include delayed nerve conduction velocity and albuminocytologic dissociation in the cerebrospinal fluid. GBS typically progresses rapidly and reaches a peak within 4 weeks of onset, and then recovers gradually. The prognosis is not always good as the disease can lead to death, incomplete recovery, and relapse. In particular, rapid progression to respiratory muscle paralysis over a short period of time is associated with a poor prognosis.

23.4.1.3 Treatment

Supportive care including mechanical ventilation for respiratory failure is significantly important. Disease modifying treatment by apheresis or IVIG has been proven superior to supportive care in several RCTs. While IVIG was reported to be as effective as apheresis in a meta-analysis [11], its precise mechanism of action is still unknown. PE combined with IVIG did not show a synergistic effect compared with PE alone or IVIG alone in an RCT [12].

23.4.2   Methods

23.4.2.1   Limited Reimbursement Under the Japanese Health Insurance System

Treatment of cases with the Hughes functional grading scale grade IV (unable to walk more than 5 m even with a walker) or V (use of mechanical ventilation) is covered by the Japanese health insurance system for up to 7 sessions per month and for up to 3 months.

23.4.2.2   Modality

IAPP with Immusorba TR-350®, which requires no replacement solution, may be recommended because IAPP demonstrated noninferiority compared to PE [13]. For PE, albumin is recommended as replacement solution because albumin offers similar efficacy with fewer complications compared to fresh frozen plasma (FFP) [14].

23.4.2.3   Treatment Schedule

A typical treatment schedule will include a total of 3–4 sessions on consecutive days or every other day for 7 days, and additional 2–4 sessions every other day in cases with insufficient recovery and symptomatic relapse. The frequency of apheresis or the target volume of plasma should be coordinated according to symptoms and IgG removal rate (aimed at 60–70 %).

It is recommended to start apheresis as early as possible within 14 days, because data suggest that starting PE within 14 days of onset, particularly within 7 days, leads to better functional recovery.

Note: Apheresis for Miller–Fischer Syndrome
Miller–Fischer syndrome is a variant form of GBS with cerebellar ataxia and external ophthalmoplegia. Although anti-ganglioside GQ1b antibodies (IgG) are present in the vast majority of patients with this form of GBS, a retrospective analysis of 50 cases revealed that removal of the autoantibodies by apheresis did not improve the cumulative probability or speed of recovery from symptoms, and that almost all patients in the study improved spontaneously with or without apheresis [15]. However, apheresis may be indicated for the treatment of a MFS subpopulation with GBS overlap.

23.5   Chronic Inflammatory Demyelinating Polyneuropathy

23.5.1   Targeted Substances and Disease Characteristics

23.5.1.1   Targeted Substances

- Autoantibodies such as anti-ganglioside GM1 antibodies (IgG)

Humoral components of the immune system including TNF-α, IFN-γ, other inflammatory cytokines, adhesive molecules, and complement components, are also thought to be involved in the disease process.

23.5.1.2   Disease Characteristics

CIDP is a multifocal neuropathy with symmetric limb weakness and sensory involvement that exhibits a slowly progressive or relapsing-remitting course over more than 2 months. Electrodiagnostic testing will show evidence of demyelination and cerebrospinal fluid analysis will demonstrate albuminocytologic dissociation. The diagnostic utility of nerve biopsy is controversial. Subtypes of CIDP include demyelinating neuropathy complicated by systemic disorders such as diabetes mellitus and systemic lupus erythematosus, and CIDP accompanied by monoclonal gammopathy of undetermined significance (see Note "Chronic Inflammatory Demyelinating Polyneuropathy associated with Monoclonal Gammopathy of Undetermined Significance").

23.5.1.3   Treatment

Several RCTs have revealed that apheresis, IVIG, and glucocorticoids are effective, while each treatment has its own advantages and disadvantages. Treatment decisions should be made based on the cost of treatment, disease type, severity of the disease, progression and remission rates, age of the patient, and risk of side effects. Apheresis is generally recommended for acute exacerbation of CIDP because rapid improvement can be expected. However, apheresis appears to be ineffective in improving chronic progressive type CIDP, sensory disturbance, or severe amyotrophy. A combination of apheresis with IVIG, glucocorticoids, and immunosuppressive agents may be considered for long-term control of disease activity.

23.5.2   Methods

23.5.2.1   Limited Reimbursement Under the Japanese Health Insurance System

The cost of treatment is reimbursed for up to 7 sessions per month and for up to 3 months under the Japanese health insurance system.

23.5.2.2   Modality

While PE has been recommended based on the results of several studies including a RCT [16], IAPP with Immusorba TR-350® and DFPP are also thought be as effective as PE as suggested in several Japanese case reports.

23.5.2.3   Treatment Schedule

A typical treatment schedule is to start with 2–3 sessions a week, continue the treatment until there is an improvement in motor function, and then gradually increase the intervals between sessions to once every 1–4 weeks.

> **Note: Chronic Inflammatory Demyelinating Polyneuropathy associated with Monoclonal Gammopathy of Undetermined Significance**
> CIDP can occur in association with a MGUS as well as a variety of other systemic illnesses. Data also show that 16–28 % of patients with a MGUS manifest polyneuropathy. While IgM MGUS is less common than non-IgM MGUS (15 % and 85 %, respectively), IgM MGUS is more common among CIDP-MGUS patients. Autoantibodies to myelin-associated glycoprotein are detected in 50 % of CIDP patients with IgM MGUS. There is a study suggesting that PE may not be as efficacious for IgM gammopathy as for IgA or IgG gammopathy [17].

23.6   Multiple Sclerosis

23.6.1   Targeted Substances and Disease Characteristics

23.6.1.1   Targeted Substances

While there are many theories about the pathogenesis of MS, no specific autoantibodies that directly cause MS have been identified to date. However, it has been speculated that apheresis has a positive impact on both humoral and cellular immunity. The following mechanisms of action have been suggested:

Humoral immunity: removal of substances implicated in MS such as autoantibodies to anti-myelin basic protein (MBP) and anti-myelin oligodendrocyte glycoprotein (MOG), serum IgG, IgM, and complement components.

Cellular immunity: suppression of antibody production through reductions in monocyte IL-1 and IL-2 production, CD4/8 ratio, and activated T cells, and an increase in the number of natural killer T cells, and activation of suppressor T cells.

23.6.1.2   Disease Characteristics

MS is an inflammatory demyelinating disease of the central nervous system with temporal and spatial dissemination of demyelinating lesions. It typically occurs in young adults and progresses gradually with cycles of relapse and remission. Visual disturbance is the common chief complaint at onset, followed by a variety of symptoms such as paralysis of limbs, cerebellar ataxia, sensory disturbance, and bladder and rectal disturbance. MS is classified according to its clinical course: relapsing-remitting MS (RRMS), primary progressive MS (PPMS), secondary progressive MS (SPMS), and progressive relapsing MS (PRMS). It has been shown that many RRMS patients will progress to SPMS at some point.

23.6.1.3   Treatment

A variety of treatments have been tried for MS of different types at different phases of the disease. Generally, interferon beta is recommended for RRMS except for periods of acute exacerbation, while various types of immunosuppressive agents have been used to treat progressive MS (PPMS and SMPS) without clear standards. A clinical trial of IVIG for MS is currently ongoing in Japan.

For the acute exacerbation phase of RRMS, while steroid pulse therapy is generally the first choice, apheresis is also recommended based on the result of an RCT showing that apheresis helped recovery from acute exacerbation and decreased the recurrence rate [18]. However, apheresis for progressive MS (PRMS and SPMS) was not found to be effective in an RCT [19]. For newly diagnosed MS, apheresis may be considered because the vast majority of MS patients start with RRMS. In refractory cases, a combination of apheresis with steroid pulse therapy and immunosuppressants may be a good option worth exploring.

23.6.2   Methods

23.6.2.1   Limited Reimbursement Under the Japanese Health Insurance System

The cost of apheresis treatment for the acute exacerbation phase of RRMS, non-responders to glucocorticoids, and patients intolerant to glucocorticoids due to side effects and other safety concerns, is reimbursed for up to 7 sessions per month and for up to 3 months.

23.6.2.2   Modality

IAPP with Immusorba TR-350® may be recommended, which is supported by a study comparing IAPP and PE showing that the IAPP group had fewer side effects while both treatments were equally effective [20]. However, DFPP or PE is recommended when IAPP is ineffective.

23.6.2.3   Treatment Schedule

A typical treatment schedule is to start every other day or twice a week and then adjust the frequency according to symptoms. It is recommended to start apheresis as early as possible for better efficacy.

Note: Apheresis for Neuromyelitis Optica
Neuromyelitis optica (NMO) or Devic disease is an inflammatory demyelinating disorder that affects the bilateral optic nerves and spinal cord. In Japan, NMO has been regarded as a variant of MS (an Asian optic-spinal form of MS) in terms of clinical course and pathological characteristics. However, IgG1 autoantibodies to aquaporin4 (AQP4) water channel have been detected from sera of NMO patients, suggesting astrocyte impairment associated with the loss of AQP4 [21]. The data support the significance of apheresis for removal of these antibodies.

References

1. Ame AN (1996) Assessment of plasmapheresis. Report of the Therapeutics and Technology Assessment Subcommittee of the American Academy of Neurology. Neurology 47 (3):840–843
2. Weinstein R (2000) Therapeutic apheresis in neurological disorders. J Clin Apher 15(1–2):74–128
3. Zinman L, Ng E, Bril V (2007) IV immunoglobulin in patients with myasthenia gravis: a randomized controlled trial. Neurology 68(11):837–841. doi:10.1212/01.wnl.0000256698.69121.45
4. Barth D, Nabavi Nouri M, Ng E, Nwe P, Bril V (2011) Comparison of IVIg and PLEX in patients with myasthenia gravis. Neurology 76(23):2017–2023. doi:10.1212/WNL.0b013e31821e5505
5. Liu JF, Wang WX, Xue J, Zhao CB, You HZ, Lu JH, Gu Y (2010) Comparing the autoantibody levels and clinical efficacy of double filtration plasmapheresis, immunoadsorption, and intravenous immunoglobulin for the treatment of late-onset myasthenia gravis. Ther Apher Dial (official peer-reviewed journal of the International Society for Apheresis, the Japanese Society for Apheresis, the Japanese Society for Dialysis Therapy) 14(2):153–160. doi:10.1111/j.1744-9987.2009.00751.x
6. Grob D, Simpson D, Mitsumoto H, Hoch B, Mokhtarian F, Bender A, Greenberg M, Koo A, Nakayama S (1995) Treatment

of myasthenia gravis by immunoadsorption of plasma. Neurology 45(2):338–344

7. Yeh JH, Chiu HC (2000) Comparison between double-filtration plasmapheresis and immunoadsorption plasmapheresis in the treatment of patients with myasthenia gravis. J Neurol 247(7): 510–513

8. Newsom-Davis J, Murray NM (1984) Plasma exchange and immunosuppressive drug treatment in the Lambert-Eaton myasthenic syndrome. Neurology 34(4):480–485

9. Nakatsuji Y, Kaido M, Sugai F, Nakamori M, Abe K, Watanabe O, Arimura K, Sakoda S (2000) Isaacs' syndrome successfully treated by immunoadsorption plasmapheresis. Acta Neurol Scand 102(4):271–273

10. Pham HP, Daniel-Johnson JA, Stotler BA, Stephens H, Schwartz J (2011) Therapeutic plasma exchange for the treatment of anti-NMDA receptor encephalitis. J Clin Apher 26(6):320–325. doi:10.1002/jca.20311

11. Hughes RA, Swan AV, van Doorn PA (2012) Intravenous immunoglobulin for Guillain-Barre syndrome. Cochrane Database Syst Rev 7:CD002063. doi:10.1002/14651858.CD002063.pub5

12. Randomised trial of plasma exchange, intravenous immunoglobulin, and combined treatments in Guillain-Barre syndrome. Plasma Exchange/Sandoglobulin Guillain-Barre Syndrome Trial Group (1997). Lancet 349 (9047):225–230

13. Diener HC, Haupt WF, Kloss TM, Rosenow F, Philipp T, Koeppen S, Vietorisz A, Study G (2001) A preliminary, randomized, multicenter study comparing intravenous immunoglobulin, plasma exchange, and immune adsorption in Guillain-Barre syndrome. Eur Neurol 46(2):107–109, doi:50777

14. Efficiency of plasma exchange in Guillain-Barre syndrome: role of replacement fluids. French Cooperative Group on Plasma Exchange in Guillain-Barre syndrome (1987). Ann Neurol 22 (6):753–761. doi:10.1002/ana.410220612

15. Mori M, Kuwabara S, Fukutake T, Hattori T (2002) Plasmapheresis and Miller Fisher syndrome: analysis of 50 consecutive cases. J Neurol Neurosurg Psychiatry 72(5): 680

16. Dyck PJ, Daube J, O'Brien P, Pineda A, Low PA, Windebank AJ, Swanson C (1986) Plasma exchange in chronic inflammatory demyelinating polyradiculoneuropathy. N Engl J Med 314(8):461–465. doi:10.1056/NEJM198602203140801

17. Dyck PJ, Low PA, Windebank AJ, Jaradeh SS, Gosselin S, Bourque P, Smith BE, Kratz KM, Karnes JL, Evans BA et al

(1991) Plasma exchange in polyneuropathy associated with monoclonal gammopathy of undetermined significance. N Engl J Med 325(21):1482–1486. doi:10.1056/NEJM199111213252105

18. Weiner HL, Dau PC, Khatri BO, Petajan JH, Birnbaum G, McQuillen MP, Fosburg MT, Feldstein M, Orav EJ (1989) Double-blind study of true vs. sham plasma exchange in patients treated with immunosuppression for acute attacks of multiple sclerosis. Neurology 39(9):1143–1149

19. The Canadian cooperative trial of cyclophosphamide and plasma exchange in progressive multiple sclerosis. The Canadian Cooperative Multiple Sclerosis Study Group (1991). Lancet 337 (8739):441–446

20. Schmitt E, von Appen K, Behm E, Kundt G, Lakner K, Meyer-Rienecker H, Palm M, Sehland D, Klinkmann H (1993) Immunoadsorption with phenylalanine-immobilized polyvinyl alcohol versus plasma exchange – a controlled pilot study in multiple sclerosis. Ther Plasmapheresis 12:239–242

21. Misu T, Fujihara K, Kakita A, Konno H, Nakamura M, Watanabe S, Takahashi T, Nakashima I, Takahashi H, Itoyama Y (2007) Loss of aquaporin 4 in lesions of neuromyelitis optica: distinction from multiple sclerosis. Brain (a journal of neurology) 130(Pt 5):1224–1234. doi:10.1093/brain/awm047

Chapter 24
Dermatological Disorders

Masao Iwagami and Kousuke Negishi

Main Points
- In severe or refractory pemphigus and pemphigoid, apheresis is performed to remove IgG autoantibodies.
- In toxic epidermal necrosis, which is often serious and life-threatening, apheresis should be considered from an early stage as a life-saving procedure.
- Infection control, IgG measurement, and the administration of fresh frozen plasma may be necessary because apheresis is often performed when the patient is in a severely immunosuppressed state.

M. Iwagami (✉)
Department of Hemodialysis & Apheresis, University Hospital,
The University of Tokyo, 7-3-1 Hongo, Bunkyo-ku, Tokyo 113-8655, Japan
e-mail: iwagami-tky@umin.ac.jp

K. Negishi
Department of Internal Medicine, Nephrology, Toshiba General Hospital,
6-3-22 Higashi-Ohi, Shinagawa-ku, Tokyo 140-8522, Japan
e-mail: knegishi-tky@umin.ac.jp

E. Noiri and N. Hanafusa (eds.), *The Concise Manual*
of Apheresis Therapy, DOI 10.1007/978-4-431-54412-8_24,
© Springer Japan 2014

24.1   Pemphigus and Pemphigoid

24.1.1   Targeted Substances and Disease Characteristics

24.1.1.1   Targeted Substances

- Specific autoantibodies of IgG class against adhesion molecules in skin tissues (Table 24.1).

24.1.1.2   Disease Characteristics

Pemphigus is an autoimmune bullous disease in which desmoglein (Dsg), an epidermal cell adhesion molecule, is targeted by autoantibodies. The disruption of intercellular adhesion leads to acantholysis and subsequent intraepidermal blister formation. In pemphigoid, autoantibodies are directed against components of the hemidesmosome as targeted antigens, e.g. bullous pemphigoid antigen 180 (BP180), resulting in subepidermal blistering. IgG antibodies to Dsg and BP180 can be detected both in the blood and as skin tissue deposits.

TABLE 24.1   Autoantigens and specific autoantibodies of autoimmune bullous diseases

	Autoantigen	Autoantibody (IgG)
Pemphigus vulgaris (PV)	Desmoglein (Dsg) 3	Anti Dsg3 antibody
Pemphigus foliaceus (PF)	Dsg1	Anti Dsg1 antibody
Bullous pemphigoid (BP)	BP180	Anti BP180 antibody
Mucous membrane pemphigoid (MMP)	BP180, laminin-5	Anti BP180 antibody, Anti laminin-5 antibody
Epidermolysis bullosa acquisita (EBA)	Type VII collagen	Anti EBA antibody

24.1.1.3   Specifics

Pemphigus Vulgaris

Pemphigus vulgaris (PV) is the most common form of pemphigus and occurs frequently in people of middle-age or older. It typically starts with painful refractory oropharyngeal mucosal erosions and ulcerations, followed by flaccid bullae and erosions involving the skin of the whole body in severe cases.

Pemphigus Foliaceus

Pemphigus foliaceus (PF) exhibits erythema with scaling and crusting, erosions, and blisters on the face, head, chest, and back. Involvement of the mucous membranes rarely occurs. PF can be induced by drugs (mostly penicillamine, captopril, or piroxicam) and neoplasms such as lymphoma.

Bullous Pemphigoid

Bullous pemphigoid (BP) is the most common form of pemphigoid and occurs frequently at age 60 or older and is characterized by erythema with pruritus and tense subepidermal blisters.

Others

Autoimmune bullous disease is a large clinical entity that includes other conditions such as mucous membrane pemphigoid (MMP) and epidermolysis bullosa acquisita (EBA).

24.1.1.4   Treatment

Oral glucocorticoids are the standard therapy, and steroid pulse therapy, immunosuppressive agents, and intravenous immunoglobulin (IVIG) are considered for severe cases. While pemphigoid lesions respond better to steroids than does pemphigus, they often require long-term exposure to immunosuppressive agents to prevent relapse. Direct removal of autoantibodies with apheresis has been proven effective, and therefore is recommended for severe cases [1]. The efficacy of apheresis on MMP and EBA has also been shown [2, 3].

24.1.2   Methods

24.1.2.1   Limited Reimbursement Under the Japanese Health Insurance System

The cost of apheresis treatment is reimbursed after a definitive diagnosis of PV, PF, or BP has been made, for cases that are refractory to other treatments, and cases for which glucocorticoids or immunosuppressive agents are not indicated due to complications or side effects. It is reimbursed for treatment frequencies of up to twice a week and for a period of up to 3 months. An additional 3 months are allowed when the disease remains moderate to severe after the initial 3 months of treatment.

24.1.2.2   Modality

There has been no clinical trial comparing plasma exchange (PE), double filtration plasmapheresis (DFPP), and immunoadsorption plasmapheresis (IAPP) in the treatment of these diseases, probably because of their low prevalence and heterogeneity. However, DFPP has been used traditionally in Japan, and IAPP also has been found effective in several case reports. When PE is performed, 5 % albumin is preferred to fresh frozen plasma (FFP) in terms of medical resource utilization and infection risk. The target volume of plasma treated is 2–2.5 L regardless of body weight for IAPP and 1–1.5 plasma volumes (PV) for DFPP and PE. PV (in liters) is calculated as $0.07 \times$ body weight $[kg] \times (1 - 0.01 \times$ hematocrit $[\%])$. Heparin is usually recommended as an anticoagulant, whereas nafamostat mesylate is a better alternative for patients with bleeding tendencies.

24.1.2.3   Treatment Schedule

A typical treatment schedule is to begin two times a week and then adjust the frequency according to symptoms and changes in antibody titers.

24.1.3   Points to Note

24.1.3.1   Hypotension

Hypotension might occur due to changes in colloid oncotic pressure and electrolytes. Therefore, when DFPP is used, the rate of albumin replacement should be controlled by continuous hematocrit monitoring (Crit-Line In-Line Monitor™ [In-Line Diagnostics, Kaysville, UT]), so that the range of blood volume change is held within a few percentages points.

24.1.3.2   Bleeding Tendency

Gamma globulins such as IgG, coagulation factors, and platelets are lost by repeated apheresis, especially when albumin is used as a replacement fluid. Replacement of these factors should be considered to manage the increased bleeding tendency.

24.1.3.3   Infection

Implementation of appropriate infection control measures such as keeping the catheter insertion point clean and changing catheters regularly every 2–3 weeks is essential when the catheter is left in place for an extended period of time.

24.1.3.4   Catheter Insertion Site

The site of catheter insertion (neck or groin) should be carefully selected because excoriation may make catheter fixation difficult.

24.2   Steven–Johnson Syndrome and Toxic Epidermal Necrolysis

24.2.1   Introduction

The diagnosis of Steven–Johnson syndrome (SJS), toxic epidermal necrolysis (TEN), and SJS/TEN overlap syndrome was proposed in 1993 according to the percentage of the body surface with skin sloughing: <10 % in SJS, >30 % in TEN, and 10–30 % in SJS/TEN [4]. In Japan, a spectrum of skin conditions with epidermal detachment and mucous membrane erosions is defined as acute-phase erythema exsudativum multiforme major (EEMM). Acute-phase EEMM includes SJS, TEN, and drug-induced hypersensitivity syndrome (DIHS) (Table 24.2), and SJS/TEN overlap syndrome is classified as TEN. Differential diagnosis is often difficult in a very early stage of the disease.

TABLE 24.2 Drugs suspected to cause toxic epidermal necrolysis based on the cases reported to the Japanese Ministry of Health, Labour and Welfare in 2009

Type of medication	Generic name
Antipyretic analgesics	Diclofenac sodium, loxoprofen sodium, acetaminophen, non-pyrine common cold remedies
Anticonvulsants	Phenobarbital, carbamazepine, zonisamide
Antibiotics	Levofloxacin, vancomycin hydrochloride, amoxicillin, piperacillin sodium
Antiulcer drugs	Famotidine
Others	Allopurinol, amlodipine besylate

24.2.2   Targeted Substances and Disease Characteristics

24.2.2.1   Targeted Substances

- Proinflammatory cytokines such as TNF-α and IFN-γ
- Soluble Fas ligand

24.2.2.2   Disease Characteristics

SJS/TEN is characterized by exudative erythema with blisters, erosions, bleeding, excoriation of mucous membranes (lips, oral cavity, eyes, nose, digestive tract, and external genitalis), and fever. Laboratory test results include increased or decreased white blood cell count, hepatic dysfunction, elevated C-reactive protein levels, renal dysfunction, hematopoietic injury, and disseminated intravascular coagulation.

Although the pathologic mechanisms of the disease are not fully understood, there are several suspected factors that may mediate apoptosis of keratinocytes, causing necrosis of the skin and mucous membranes: a cytolytic protein called granulysin produced by cytotoxic T lymphocytes and natural killer cells, proinflammatory cytokines such as TNF-α and IFN-γ, and soluble Fas ligand.

24.2.2.3   Treatment

After discontinuation of causative drugs, systemic glucocorticoids are commonly administered. In severe cases, steroid pulse therapy and IVIG are considered. Apheresis has been proven effective in several studies [5]. PE or DFPP is considered in the early stages of the disease when glucocorticoids are ineffective or cannot be used for safety reasons such as an increased risk of infection. Early diagnosis and treatment are important to reduce mortality and sequelae such as pulmonary obstructive disorders and blindness.

24.2.3   Methods

24.2.3.1   Limited Reimbursement Under the Japanese Health Insurance System

The cost of apheresis treatment for TEN and SJS is reimbursed for up to eight sessions.

24.2.3.2   Modality

Both PE and DFPP are covered by the Japanese health insurance system. It is generally thought that PE can remove a greater amount of cytokines and therefore improve symptoms more effectively than DFPP. However, PE has disadvantages such as high costs, FFP-associated infection, production of irregular antibodies, and allergic reactions. Nafamostat mesylate is usually recommended as an anticoagulant because SJS/TEN patients often have bleeding tendencies.

24.2.3.3   Treatment Schedule

A typical treatment schedule is to begin with daily or every-other-day sessions, and then adjust the frequency according to changes in symptoms.

24.2.4   Points to Note

Same as pemphigus and pemphigoid (see Sect. 24.1.3).

References

1. Takamori K, Yamada H, Morioka S, Ogawa H (1993) Long term remission successfully achieved in severe types of pemphigus vulgaris and bullous pemphigoid by the use of plasmapheresis. Eur J Dermatol 3:433–437

2. Hashimoto Y, Suga Y, Yoshiike T, Hashimoto T, Takamori K (2000) A case of antiepiligrin cicatricial pemphigoid successfully treated by plasmapheresis. Dermatology 201(1):58–60. doi:10.1159/000018433

3. Kubisch I, Diessenbacher P, Schmidt E, Gollnick H, Leverkus M (2010) Premonitory epidermolysis bullosa acquisita mimicking eyelid dermatitis: successful treatment with rituximab and protein A immunoapheresis. Am J Clin Dermatol 11(4):289–293. doi:10.2165/11533210-000000000-00000

4. Bastuji-Garin S, Rzany B, Stern RS, Shear NH, Naldi L, Roujeau JC (1993) Clinical classification of cases of toxic epidermal necrolysis, Stevens-Johnson syndrome, and erythema multiforme. Arch Dermatol 129(1):92–96

5. Yamada H, Takamori K (2008) Status of plasmapheresis for the treatment of toxic epidermal necrolysis in Japan. Ther Apher Dial (official peer-reviewed journal of the International Society for Apheresis, the Japanese Society for Apheresis, the Japanese Society for Dialysis Therapy) 12(5):355–359. doi:10.1111/j.1744-9987.2008.00609.x

Chapter 25
Kidney Diseases

Masao Iwagami and Kousuke Negishi

Main Points
- LDL apheresis for the treatment of focal segmental glomerulosclerosis (FSGS) in patients with refractory nephrotic syndrome is effective and may increase sensitivity to glucocorticoids and cyclosporine.
- Apheresis should be considered for patients with severe rapidly progressive glomerulonephritis (RPGN) to preserve their remaining renal function.

M. Iwagami (✉)
Department of Internal Medicine, Toshiba General Hospital,
7-3-1 Hongo, Bunkyo-ku, Tokyo 113-8655, Japan
e-mail: iwagami-tky@umin.ac.jp

K. Negishi
Department of Internal Medicine, Nephrology, Toshiba General Hospital,
6-3-22 Higashi-Ohi, Shinagawa-ku, Tokyo 140-8522, Japan
e-mail: knegishi-tky@umin.ac.jp

E. Noiri and N. Hanafusa (eds.), *The Concise Manual*
of Apheresis Therapy, DOI 10.1007/978-4-431-54412-8_25,
© Springer Japan 2014

25.1 Nephrotic Syndrome (NS)

25.1.1 Introduction

Nephrotic syndrome (NS) is a condition characterized by heavy proteinuria of more than 3.5 g/day and hypoalbuminemia of <3.0 g/dL. Edema and hyperlipidemia are observed frequently in patients with NS. NS is classified as primary NS and secondary NS. The Japan Kidney Disease Registry revealed that among 1,197 patients with NS registered from 2007 to 2009, the proportion with primary NS was 66.2 %, followed by secondary NS due to diabetes mellitus and lupus nephritis accounting for 10.7 % and 4.5 %, respectively [1]. Table 25.1 shows the distribution of histopathologic subtypes of primary NS in 732 cases from the registry. About 20 % of patients with NS have refractory disease with persistent proteinuria of more than 1 g/day despite 6 months of standard therapy with glucocorticoids and immunosuppressive agents. Focal segmental glomerulosclerosis (FSGS) is often associated with NS that is resistant to treatment. The cost of apheresis treatment for FSGS has been reimbursed under the Japanese health insurance system based on several studies demonstrating its efficacy.

25.1.2 Focal Segmental Glomerulosclerosis

25.1.2.1 Targeted Substances and Disease Characteristics

Targeted Substances

Low density lipoprotein (LDL), lipoprotein (a), very low density lipoprotein (VLDL), and intermediate density lipoprotein (IDL) are targets of apheresis therapy in patients with FSGS.

Disease Characteristics

FSGS is classified as primary or idiopathic, with no identified cause, and secondary FSGS, with an identified underlying cause such as obesity or HIV infection. Primary FSGS

TABLE 25.1 Distribution of histopathologic subtypes of primary nephrotic syndrome (NS) in 732 cases registered in the Japan Kidney Disease Registry from 2007 to 2009 [1]

Histopathologic subtypes	Proportion (%)
Minimal change disease	38.7
Membranous nephropathy	37.8
Focal segmental glomerulosclerosis	11.1
Membranoproliferative glomerulonephritis (type I and type III)	6.6
Mesangial proliferative glomerulonephritis	2.9
Crescentic glomerulonephritis	1.4
Others	1.5

frequently occurs at a young age. FSGS accounts for approximately 50 % of refractory NS in children and 20 % of that in adults. FSGS often develops suddenly, with proteinuria of more than 10 g/day, systemic edema, and severe hyperlipidemia, and typically follows a progressive course to endstage renal disease. While it is sometimes difficult to differentiate FSGS from minimal change disease (MCD), patients with FSGS often have a high fractional urinary excretion of high-molecular-weight proteins such as IgG and a poor response to glucocorticoids compared to findings for patients with MCD. FSGS is pathologically classified into five types: Classic FSGS, collapsing variant, tip variant, perihilar variant, and cellular variant. Treatment response and renal prognosis appear to vary among these types.

Treatment

Glucocorticoids are recommended for initial remission induction therapy. A combination of cyclosporine and low-dose glucocorticoids is recommended for patients with steroid-resistant disease. LDL apheresis may be considered for patients with refractory NS, as it has been shown to work through a variety of mechanisms, including serum cholesterol reduction, recovery of platelet function and the coagulation-fibrinolysis system, suppression of lipid mediator production in the kidney, and prevention of macrophage infiltration into glomeruli. Reduction of serum cholesterol also appears to improve responsiveness to glucocorticoids and cyclosporine.

A retrospective survey revealed that FSGS patients treated with LDL apheresis had favorable short- and long-term outcomes [2]. Long-term effects of LDL apheresis are currently being evaluated in the Prospective Observational Survey on the Long-Term Effects of LDL Apheresis on the Drug Resistant Nephrotic Syndrome (POLARIS) survey. In the study, 51.9 % of recruited patients achieved complete or incomplete remission with normalized serum protein levels 1 month after LDL-apheresis. Patients treated with LDL apheresis within 8 weeks from NS onset were more responsive [3]. LDL apheresis was also reported to be effective in children with steroid-resistant primary FSGS [4].

25.1.2.2   Methods

Limited Reimbursement Under the Japanese Health Insurance System

The cost of apheresis treatment for FSGS in patients with a persistent nephrotic condition and serum total cholesterol greater than 250 mg/dL despite conventional therapies is reimbursed for up to 7 sessions per month and for up to 3 months.

Modality

Plasma adsorption (PA) with a dextran sulfate column is the first choice for apheresis because the negatively charged dextran sulfate can adsorb LDL, lipoprotein (a), VLDL, and IDL via the positively charged apolipoprotein B. The cost of double filtration plasmapheresis (DFPP) is also reimbursed and may be effective when PA does not work. The target volume of treated plasma is 3–5 L with PA and 2–4 L with DFPP. Heparin usually is recommended as an anticoagulant, whereas nafamostat mesylate is preferred for patients at high risk of bleeding.

Treatment Schedule

A typical treatment schedule consists of 2 sessions per week for 6 weeks or 2 sessions per week for 3 weeks followed by 1 session per week for 6 weeks (9 weeks in total).

Points to Note

See Sect. 30.4

25.1.3   Apheresis for Other NS

LDL apheresis or cytapheresis for primary refractory NS, including membranous nephropathy and MCD, has been investigated but its efficacy has not yet been established. Proven effective treatments for secondary NS include plasma exchange (PE) for patients with lupus nephritis, PE for patients with multiple myeloma, and cryofiltration for those with cryoglobulinemia. The effectiveness of LDL apheresis has also been demonstrated for patients with diabetic nephropathy with NS [5]. Further studies of apheresis for the treatment of NS are awaited.

> **Note: Recurrence of FSGS After Kidney Transplantation**
> Approximately 30 % of patients with primary FSGS have an early recurrence with high-grade proteinuria after kidney transplantation. PE has been shown to decrease proteinuria in such cases, indicating that some circulating factors (CFs) may increase glomerular permeability. Serum soluble urokinase receptor (suPAR) has been identified as a CF that activates podocyte $\beta 3$ integrin to trigger FSGS [6]. Because SuPAR is 20–50 kDa in size (depending on the degree of modification such as glycosylation) and does not have a high affinity to albumin, it can be removed by apheresis, resulting in reduction of proteinuria. Therefore, apheresis is expected to play an increasingly important role in the treatment of FSGS.

25.2   Rapidly Progressive Glomerulonephritis (RPGN)

25.2.1   Introduction

Rapidly progressive glomerulonephritis (RPGN) is a clinical syndrome characterized by rapidly progressive loss of renal function over weeks or months and urinalysis findings indicative of glomerulonephritis, including hematuria, proteinuria, granular casts, and erythrocyte casts. The diagnosis usually is confirmed by renal biopsy showing glomerular crescent formation. Systemic symptoms and results of serum biomarker analysis should also be considered. The distribution of clinical and pathological diagnoses in 567 Japanese cases with RPGN is shown in Table 25.2.

25.2.2   Targeted Substances and Disease Characteristics

25.2.2.1   Targeted Substances

Autoantibodies directed against the glomerular basement membrane (GBM), anti-neutrophil cytoplasmic antibodies (ANCA) directed against myeloperoxidase (MPO) and proteinase-3 (PR3) often are associated with RPGN and removed with apheresis. Removal of other factors such as proinflammatory cytokines, complement, and immune complexes may also lead to improvement of RPGN.

25.2.2.2   Disease Characteristics

RPGN occurs frequently in middle-aged and older people, sometimes triggered by infections. Initial signs and symptoms include fatigue, fever, anorexia, edema, bubbles in the urine related to proteinuria, hematuria, nausea, and weight loss.

TABLE 25.2 Distribution of clinical and pathological diagnoses in 567 cases with rapidly progressive glomerulonephritis (RPGN) reported in the Japanese national questionnaire survey from 2002 to 2007 [7]

Clinical and pathological diagnosis	Proportion (%)
Primary	
Pauci-immune crescentic glomerulonephritis	43.9
Anti-glomerular basement membrane (anti-GBM) crescentic glomerulonephritis	3.9
Unclassifiable primary crescentic glomerulonephritis	2.1
IgA nephropathy with crescentic formation	1.6
Mixed type crescentic glomerulonephritis	1.2
Immune complex type crescentic glomerulonephritis	1.1
Membranoproliferative glomerulonephritis with crescentic formation	0.7
Systemic	
Microscopic polyangiitis	22.8
Wegener's granulomatosis	2.5
Purpura nephritis	2.3
Systemic lupus erythematosus	1.9
Other systemic disorders	1.6
Goodpasture syndrome	1.4
Rheumatoid arthritis	0.7
Cryoglobulinemia	0.7
Other forms of necrotizing angiitis	0.7
Infectious	
Other infectious diseases	0.9
Infectious endocarditis	0.5
Poststreptococcal glomerulonephritis	<0.1
Other	1.6
Unknown	6.9

Extra-renal symptoms include joint pain, muscle pain, hemoptysis, purpura, and melena. Disease onset has shifted to older individuals: RPGN, 64.7 ± 16.6 years (mean ± SD), range 1–93 years; pauci-immune type crescentic GN 67.3 ± 13.1 (mean ± SD), range 1–92. Elderly patients over 80 years of age are not rare in Japan [7]. Laboratory test results show the presence of autoantibodies such as MPO-ANCA, PR3-ANCA, or anti-GBM antibody. Antibody titers, urinalysis results, and serum creatinine and C-reactive protein (CRP) levels often correlate with disease activity.

Pathologic features include crescent formation and breaks in the glomerular capillary wall and the GBM. Crescentic glomerulonephritis is classified into three types: (1) anti-GBM type characterized by linear deposition of IgG and C3 on the GBM; (2) immune complex type with granular deposition of IgG and C3 on the mesangium and the GBM; and (3) pauci-immune type with no deposition of immunoglobulin or complement.

25.2.2.3   Treatment

While the treatment strategy depends on the type of RPGN, glucocorticoids and immunosuppressive agents such as cyclophosphamide are the mainstay of treatment. Early diagnosis and treatment are important because of high mortality rates and rapid progression to endstage renal disease (ESRD).

Several studies have evaluated the efficacy of apheresis for RPGN. Apheresis is recommended for anti-GBM antibody associated RPGN based on reports of its effectiveness for restoring renal function even in patients with high serum creatinine levels [8]. The European Vasculitis Study Group (EUVAS) showed that for patients with ANCA-associated RPGN receiving oral prednisolone and oral cyclophosphamide, the addition of PE (7 sessions within 14 days) was more effective for achieving renal recovery than adjunctive therapy with intravenous methylprednisolone (1,000 mg for 3 days). Survival and severe adverse event rates were similar in both groups [9]. However, plasmapheresis provided no long-term benefit over intravenous methylprednisolone (median follow-up period of 4 years) [10]. A meta-analysis of nine trials (387 patients) concluded that PE decreased the relative risk for ESRD in patients with renal vasculitis and idiopathic RPGN, whereas the relative risk for death was not significantly different [11]. The Plasma Exchange and Glucocorticoids for Treatment of Anti-Neutrophil Cytoplasmic Antibody (ANCA)—Associated Vasculitis (PEXIVAS) study is now in progress.

25.2.3   Methods

25.2.3.1   Limited Reimbursement Under the Japanese Health Insurance System

At the current time, the cost of apheresis treatment for RPGN is not reimbursed. However, apheresis should be considered, based on the aforementioned evidence, for patients with severe RPGN.

25.2.3.2   Modality

PE is the first choice, and DFPP is also recommended for the treatment of RPGN. Cytapheresis may be effective for MPO-ANCA associated vasculitis (see **Note "The Effect of Cytapheresis on MPO-ANCA Associated Vasculitis"**).

25.2.3.3   Treatment Schedule

A typical treatment schedule begins with two to three treatments per week with subsequent adjustments of the frequency according to symptoms and changes in laboratory parameters, such as antibody titers and CRP.

Note: The Effect of Cytapheresis on MPO-ANCA Associated Vasculitis

Cytapheresis may be effective for the treatment of MPO-ANCA associated vasculitis. Plasma levels of TNF-α, a proinflammatory cytokine, are known to increase in MPO-ANCA associated vasculitis, which has been treated with an anti-TNF-α antibody (infliximab). Cytapheresis has been reported to increase plasma levels of soluble tumor necrosis factor receptors (sTNFR1, sTNFR2), which act as TNF-antagonists, and to decrease the number of degranulated granulocytes expressing CD63, an inflammatory mediator [12]. Further studies are awaited to examine the clinical impact of cytapheresis in patients with MPO-ANCA associated vasculitis.

References

1. Imai E (2011) Guidelines for the treatment of nephrotic syndrome. Nihon Jinzou Gakkai Shi 53(2):78–122
2. Muso E, Mune M, Yorioka N, Nishizawa Y, Hirano T, Hattori M, Sugiyama S, Watanabe T, Kimura K, Yokoyama H, Sato H, Saito T (2007) Beneficial effect of low-density lipoprotein apheresis (LDL-A) on refractory nephrotic syndrome (NS) due to focal glomerulo-sclerosis (FGS). Clinical nephrology 67(6):341–344
3. Muso E, Saito T (2013 Abstract) Comparison of the clinical efficacy of LDL apheresis for the drug resistant nephrotic syndrome caused by focal segmental glomerulosclerosis (FGS) and non FGS in the POLARIS study. The World Congress of Nephrology 2013 abstract SA246 http://www.abstracts2view.com/wcn/view.php?nu=WCN13L_977
4. Hattori M, Chikamoto H, Akioka Y, Nakakura H, Ogino D, Matsunaga A, Fukazawa A, Miyakawa S, Khono M, Kawaguchi H, Ito K (2003) A combined low-density lipoprotein apheresis and prednisone therapy for steroid-resistant primary focal segmental glomerulosclerosis in children. Am J Kidney Dis (the official journal of the National Kidney Foundation) 42(6):1121–1130
5. Nakamura T, Kawagoe Y, Ogawa H, Ueda Y, Hara M, Shimada N, Ebihara I, Koide H (2005) Effect of low-density lipoprotein apheresis on urinary protein and podocyte excretion in patients with nephrotic

syndrome due to diabetic nephropathy. Am J Kidney Dis (the official journal of the National Kidney Foundation) 45(1):48–53

6. Wei C, El Hindi S, Li J, Fornoni A, Goes N, Sageshima J, Maiguel D, Karumanchi SA, Yap HK, Saleem M, Zhang Q, Nikolic B, Chaudhuri A, Daftarian P, Salido E, Torres A, Salifu M, Sarwal MM, Schaefer F, Morath C, Schwenger V, Zeier M, Gupta V, Roth D, Rastaldi MP, Burke G, Ruiz P, Reiser J (2011) Circulating urokinase receptor as a cause of focal segmental glomerulosclerosis. Nature medicine 17(8):952–960. doi:10.1038/nm.2411

7. Koyama A, Yamagata K, Makino H, Arimura Y, Wada T, Nitta K, Nihei H, Muso E, Taguma Y, Shigematsu H, Sakai H, Tomino Y, Matsuo S, Japan RRG (2009) A nationwide survey of rapidly progressive glomerulonephritis in Japan: etiology, prognosis and treatment diversity. Clinical and experimental nephrology 13(6):633–650. doi:10.1007/s10157-009-0201-7

8. Levy JB, Turner AN, Rees AJ, Pusey CD (2001) Long-term outcome of anti-glomerular basement membrane antibody disease treated with plasma exchange and immunosuppression. Annals of internal medicine 134(11):1033–1042

9. Jayne DR, Gaskin G, Rasmussen N, Abramowicz D, Ferrario F, Guillevin L, Mirapeix E, Savage CO, Sinico RA, Stegeman CA, Westman KW, van der Woude FJ, de Lind van Wijngaarden RA, Pusey CD, European Vasculitis Study G (2007) Randomized trial of plasma exchange or high-dosage methylprednisolone as adjunctive therapy for severe renal vasculitis. J Am Soc Nephrol 18 (7):2180–2188. doi: 10.1681/ASN.2007010090

10. Walsh M, Casian A, Flossmann O, Westman K, Höglund P, Pusey C, Jayne DR (2013) Long-term follow-up of patients with severe ANCA-associated vasculitis comparing plasma exchange to intravenous methylprednisolone treatment is unclear. Kidney International advance online publication 24 April 2013 doi: 10.1038/ki.2013.131

11. Walsh M, Catapano F, Szpirt W, Thorlund K, Bruchfeld A, Guillevin L, Haubitz M, Merkel PA, Peh CA, Pusey C, Jayne D (2011) Plasma exchange for renal vasculitis and idiopathic rapidly progressive glomerulonephritis: a meta-analysis. Am J Kidney Dis (the official journal of the National Kidney Foundation) 57(4):566–574. doi:10.1053/j.ajkd.2010.10.049

12. Hasegawa M, Nishii C, Kabutan N, Kato M, Ohashi A, Nakai S, Murakami K, Tomita M, Nabeshima K, Hiki Y, Oshima H, Sugiyama S (2007) Effects of cytapheresis on tumor necrosis factor receptor and on expression of CD63 in myeloperoxidase–antineutrophil cytoplasmic autoantibody-associated vasculitis. Ther Apher Dial (official peer-reviewed journal of the International Society for Apheresis, the Japanese Society for Apheresis, the Japanese Society for Dialysis Therapy) 11(5):337–340. doi:10.1111/j.1744-9987.2007.00496.x

Chapter 26
Rheumatoid Arthritis and Collagen Diseases

Hiroko Kanda

Main Points

Rheumatoid Arthritis

- Therapeutic apheresis is used for the treatment of rheumatoid arthritis that is resistant to pharmacologic treatments.
- Therapeutic apheresis is performed to remove infiltrating activated T cells, B cells, neutrophils, and monocytes in patients with rheumatoid arthritis.
- Filtration leukocytapheresis (LCAP) has dose-dependent effects.

Malignant Rheumatoid Arthritis

- Therapeutic apheresis is used in addition to pharmacotherapy with glucocorticoids or immunosuppressive agents.

H. Kanda (✉)
Department of Allergy and Rheumatology, University Hospital,
The University of Tokyo, 7-3-1 Hongo, Bunkyo-ku, Tokyo 113-8655, Japan
e-mail: hkanda-tky@umin.ac.jp

E. Noiri and N. Hanafusa (eds.), *The Concise Manual of Apheresis Therapy*, DOI 10.1007/978-4-431-54412-8_26,
© Springer Japan 2014

- Immunocomplex (IC) and activated complement are removed by therapeutic apheresis.
- Plasma exchange (PE), double filtration plasmapheresis (DFPP), cryofiltration, or immunoadsorption plasmapheresis (IAPP) are chosen based on the disease status of each patient.

Systemic Lupus Erythematosus
- Therapeutic apheresis therapy is used for the treatment of systemic lupus erythematosus (SLE) that is associated with severe organ damage despite treatment with glucocorticoids or immunosuppressive agents.
- Therapeutic apheresis removes IC and autoantibodies.
- Plasma exchange (PE), double filtration plasmapheresis (DFPP), cryofiltration, or immunoadsorption plasmapheresis (IAPP) are chosen based on the disease status of each patient.

Antiphospholipid Syndrome
- Therapeutic apheresis is used for the treatment of antiphospholipid syndrome (APS) with severe thrombotic complications leading to multi-organ damage.
- PE or IAPP is performed to remove autoantibodies and improve disorders of thrombosis and fibrinolysis.
- IAPP is repeated once a week until delivery in pregnant APS patients with recurrent spontaneous abortion despite the use of antiplatelet or anticoagulant therapy.

ANCA-Associated Vasculitis
- Therapeutic apheresis is performed for patients with ANCA-associated vasculitis that is resistant to a combination of glucocorticoids and immunosuppressive agents and is complicated with rapidly progressive glomerulonephritis (RPGN) or pulmonary bleeding.
- PE removes autoantibodies.

26.1   Rheumatoid Arthritis

26.1.1   Introduction

LCAP is approved as a treatment for patients with rheumatoid arthritis (RA) who are resistant to multidrug therapy [glucocorticoids, disease modifying antirheumatic drugs (DMARDs)].

26.1.2   Targets and Pathology

26.1.2.1   Targets

Activated leukocytes are the target of LCAP for the treatment of RA.

26.1.2.2   Pathology

Patients with RA present with polyarthritis caused by an immunologic disorder. Naïve T cells differentiate into memory T cells after interaction with certain antigens, migrate to joint synovium, and activate monocytes. Activated monocytes secrete various cytokines, consequently joints were damaged.

26.1.3   Efficacy

The efficacy of LCAP therapy is maintained for about 2 months. The American College of Rheumatology (ACR) core set and the European League Against Rheumatism (EULAR) 28-joint disease activity score (DAS28)-C-reactive protein (CRP) were used for assessment of efficacy. When 3 L of blood were filtered with a leukocyte removal column, 60–70 % of the patients had an ACR 20 % response and 20–30 % of the patients had an ACR 50 % response [1]. When 5 L of blood were filtered with a leukocyte removal column, 78 % of the patients had an ACR 20 % response and

44 % of the patients had an ACR 50 % response. Moderate or good DAS28-CRP responses were achieved in 50–60 % of the patients [2–4].

26.1.4   Methods

26.1.4.1   Insurance Restriction

LCAP is approved for the treatment of RA in patients with more than six swollen joints, erythrocyte sedimentation rate (ESR) of more than 50 mm/h, or CRP level more than 3 mg/dL, associated with systemic symptoms such as fatigue, low-grade fever, and acute progressive polyarthritis, and resistance to multi-drug therapy. The approved schedule of LCAP treatments is once a week for 5 consecutive weeks.

26.1.4.2   Modality

CS-100 Cellsorba® is a leukocyte removal column equipped with a fiber filter for the filtration of a total of 3 L of blood. CS-180 Cellsorba® is used for the filtration of a total of 5 L of blood.

26.1.4.3   Frequency

LCAP is performed once a week for 5 consecutive weeks.

26.1.4.4   Response Indicators

CRP, ESR, and matrix metalloproteinase-3 (MMP-3) levels are used as indicators of response to treatment.

26.1.5   Points to Note

26.1.5.1   Start-Up

LCAP should be used with caution in patients with leukopenia (white blood cells <3,000/mm^3), anemia (hemoglobin

<10 g/dL), or thrombocytopenia (platelets $<100 \times 10^3/mm^3$) because the procedure may induce cytopenia. Angiotensin-converting enzyme (ACE) inhibitors should be discontinued more than 1 week prior to starting LCAP, because of the risk of hypotension induced by LCAP in patients taking ACE inhibitors, probably due to an accumulation of bradykinin.

26.1.5.2   Other Complications

Other potential complications of LCAP include hypotension, nausea, and transient anemia, but these generally are not severe.

26.2   Malignant Rheumatoid Arthritis

26.2.1   Introduction

Malignant rheumatoid arthritis (MRA) is RA complicated with vasculitis. The symptoms of vasculitis include cutaneous ulcers/infarctions/necrosis, mononeuritis multiplex, pericarditis, coronary vasculitis, pulmonary vasculitis, episcleritis, and other symptoms of systemic vasculitis, which often are refractory and severe. Apheresis therapy for MRA is covered by insurance in Japan.

26.2.2   Targets and Pathology

26.2.2.1   Targets

IC, complement, and cytokines are targets of apheresis in patients with MRA.

26.2.2.2   Pathology

MRA is associated with severe extra-articular vasculitis in addition to the typical manifestations of RA. Circulating IC composed of rheumatoid factor (RF) and antigen is deposited on vascular walls, inducing complement and neutrophil activation, increased production of cytokines, and tissue damage.

26.2.3   Efficacy

Apheresis therapy has been reported to be effective for the treatment of MRA; however, there have been no randomized controlled trials of its use in patients with MRA.

26.2.4   Methods

26.2.4.1   Insurance Restriction

Therapeutic apheresis is approved in Japan for patients with MRA and severe vasculitis that is resistant to standard treatments. DFPP or IAPP is performed once a week or less frequently. Apheresis can be repeated according to its efficacy.

26.2.4.2   Modality

Only DFPP or IAPP are covered by insurance, but PE and cryofiltration are also used in the clinical setting. PH-350 Immusorba®, a column with phenylalanine ligand, is used for IAPP.

26.2.4.3   Frequency of Treatment

Approximately 2–3 L of plasma are processed during each treatment session. Initially, apheresis is performed two or three times per week. The treatment interval may be extended to two to four times per month according to clinical efficacy. This strategy is included in the 2002 guideline for the treatment of refractory vasculitis [5].

26.2.4.4   Response Indicators

CRP, ESR, complement, white blood cells (WBCs), IC (Clq), and RF are used as indicators of response to therapy.

26.2.5   Points to Note

> **Note**
> Recently, LCAP has been reported to be effective for cutaneous ulcers in patients with MRA.

26.3   Systemic Lupus Erythematosus

26.3.1   Introduction

Systemic lupus erythematosus (SLE) is a chronic inflammatory disease caused by immunologic abnormalities; it is diagnosed according to the diagnostic criteria proposed by the ACR. Therapeutic apheresis is used to treat patients with SLE that is resistant to multi-drug therapy or who have severe organ dysfunction.

26.3.2   Targets and Pathology

26.3.2.1   Targets

IC and auto-antibodies [anti-double-strand (ds) DNA antibodies, etc.] are targeted for removal in patients with SLE.

26.3.2.2   Pathology

Environmental factors (e.g., ultraviolet light, stress, infection, estrogen) in addition to the presence of susceptibility genes (e.g., *FCGR2A, PTPN22, PDCD1*) trigger the development of the pathogenic autoantibodies and IC in patients with SLE. Autoantibodies and IC adhere to vessel walls, promoting complement activation, and cytokine production, resulting in tissue damage.

26.3.3   Efficacy

A randomized controlled trial (RCT) compared a standard-therapy regimen of glucocorticoids and oral cyclophosph-amide (CY) with a regimen of standard therapy plus PE for proliferative lupus nephritis (LN) [6]. Treatment with PE plus a standard regimen was associated with a significantly more rapid reduction in serum concentrations of antibodies against dsDNA and cryoglobulins during the initial weeks of therapy; however, the combined treatment did not result in improved long-term clinical outcomes at 300 weeks [6]. The addition of PE to glucocorticoid therapy and intravenous CY (IVCY) was also effective for inducing faster remission in patients with proliferative LN, but it was not superior to conventional therapy at long-term follow-up [7, 8]. However, in a 5-year retrospective evaluation, the combination of PE and IVCY resulted in superior LN complete remission rates and mini-mized the risk of relapse to impaired renal function com-pared with results for PE or IVCY [9].

A recent small RCT comparing PE and IAPP as adjunc-tive therapy reported that both treatments were equally well tolerated and equally effective in patients with proliferative LN [10]. PE and synchronized PE-IVCY have been shown to be effective for the inhibition of early brain damage in patients with neuropsychiatric SLE (NPSLE) [11]. Table 26.1 shows the manifestations in patients with SLE that may respond to therapeutic apheresis [12].

26.3.4   Methods

26.3.4.1   Insurance Restriction

Therapeutic apheresis is approved for the treatment of patients with glucocorticoid-resistant SLE with hypocomple-mentemia (CH50 $\leq$20 U or C3 $\leq$40 mg/dL), extremely high anti-dsDNA antibody levels, and proliferative LN or NPSLE. Patients are treated with DFPP or IAPP a maximum of four times a month. Patients with SLE complicated by thrombotic thrombocytopenic purpura (TTP) can be treated with PE a maximum of three times a week for 3 months.

TABLE 26.1 Clinical manifestations of SLE effected by therapeutic apheresis

1	Active lupus nephritis (diffuse proliperative glomerulonephritis, rapidly progressive glomerulonephritis, nephrotic syndrome etc.)
2	Neurologic manifestations (seizures, dystonia, psychosis, encephalopathy etc.)
3	Serositis (pericarditis, pleuritis etc.)
4	Cutaneous lesions (ulcers etc.)
5	Interstitial pneumonitis pulmonary bleeding
6	Generalized vasculitis
7	Thrombocytopenia
8	Hemolytic anemia, aplastic anemia
9	Hemophagocytsis
10	Thrombotic thrombocytopenic purpura
11	Antiphospholipid syndrome
12	Hereditary angioneurotic edema
13	Habitual abortion

26.3.4.2 Modality

(a) PE is used for patients with complicated TTP, hemophago-cytosis, or multiple organ failure.

(b) DFPP primarily is used for patients with secondary cryo-globulinemia, hyperviscosity, cutaneous lesions, or neuro-logic symptoms.

(c) IAPP can be performed with the Cellsorba® column, which has a dextran sulfate ligand, or with the Immusorba® column, which has a phenylalanine ligand. The Cellsorba® column primarily removes IC and anti-DNA antibodies via an electrostatic interaction, while the Immusorba® column primarily removes, anti-cardiolipin antibodies via a hydrophobic interaction. IAPP can be used for younger patients or pregnant women, because it requires no blood products and is not associated with transfusion-transmit-ted infections.

(d) Cryofiltration is mainly used for patients with secondary cryoglobulinemia.

26.3.4.3   Frequency

Approximately 2–4 L of plasma are processed during each treatment session. Apheresis is initially performed two or three times a week. The treatment interval may be extended to two to seven times per month, according to clinical efficacy of the treatments.

26.3.4.4   Response Indicators

Complement, anti-DNA antibodies, IC (C1q), CRP, and ESR are indicators of response.

26.3.5   Points to Note

Refer to each section on apheresis.

Note: Prevention of Neonatal Conduction Failure by IAPP

Neonatal lupus is caused by transplacental passage of maternal anti-SS-A and/or anti-SS-B antibodies. The frequency of congenital heart block in infants born to mothers with these antibodies was 2 %. The maternal IgG antibodies gain access to the fetal circulation via active placental transfer (which increases after week 16 of gestation) after the fetal heart has reached functional maturity (by week 16). Damage to the cardiac electroconduction system can progress through various stages to complete atrioventricular block, most often detected between 18 and 24 weeks gestation. To prevent fetal conduction failure, pregnant women with highly elevated levels of SSA-antibodies and/or a positive history of clinical complications may be treated with IAPP [13].

26.4   Antiphospholipid Syndrome

26.4.1   Introduction

APS is characterized by the presence of antiphospholipid antibodies (aPL) and thrombosis; it is diagnosed according to the APS classification criteria [14]. Therapeutic apheresis is performed in patients with treatment-resistant catastrophic APS (CAPS), which is characterized by multiple vascular occlusive events, usually affecting small vessels and developing over a short period of time. Apheresis is also performed in patients who have had recurrent spontaneous abortions.

26.4.2   Targets and Pathology

26.4.2.1   Targets

Apheresis for APS targets aPL and cytokines.

26.4.2.2   Pathology

Antiphospholipid antibodies are directed against plasma proteins bound to anionic phospholipids and include anticardiolipin antibodies, antibodies to β2 glycoprotein-I (β2 GPI), lupus anticoagulant (LA), and others. The antiphospholipid antibody β2 GPI dimmer activates the complement cascade, induces adhesion molecule expression, and activates monocytes and platelets, resulting in the release of proinflammatory mediators and induction of thrombosis.

26.4.3   Efficacy

Therapeutic apheresis for APS has not been studied in RCTs. CAPS is associated with a 50 % mortality rate; however, the mortality rate has been reduced to 30 % over the past 5 years by intensive therapies including PE and treatment with anticoagulants, glucocorticoids, and intravenous immunoglobulin

[15]. Pregnant women with APS often are treated prophylactically with a combination of heparin and low-dose aspirin or aspirin, but live births cannot be achieved in 20–30 % of patients. Adding prophylactic treatment with PE or IAPP may improve the live birth rate [16, 17].

26.4.4   Methods

26.4.4.1   Insurance Restriction

Therapeutic apheresis is not approved for APS.

26.4.4.2   Modality

(a) IAPP : Cellsorba® with dextran sulfate ligand is used for IAPP.
(b) DFPP
(c) PE

26.4.4.3   Frequency

PE is preferentially used for patients with CAPS. Treatments are initially given two or three times a week. The treatment interval is extended to two to four times per month according to the clinical response.
IAPP is used for pregnant women with APS. IAPP is started in the sixth to eighth week of pregnancy and repeated once a week until delivery.

26.4.4.4   Response Indicators

Platelet count and aPL levels are used as indicators of response.

26.4.5   Points to Note

Patients with thrombocytopenia and a bleeding tendency should be treated with nafamostat mesylate (Futhan®) for anticoagulation during apheresis.

For pregnant patients treated with IAPP, the blood flow rate should be less than 50 mL/min to maintain the placental blood flow.

26.5   ANCA-Associated Vasculitis

26.5.1   Introduction

ANCA-associated vasculitis (AAV) involves small- to medium-sized blood vessels. AAV is classified into three heterogeneous syndromes: granulomatosis with polyangiitis (GPA); microscopic polyangiitis (MPA); and the Churg–Strauss syndrome (CSS). The relevant target antigens of ANCA are proteinase 3 (PR3) and myeloperoxidase (MPO). Antibodies specific for PR3 and MPO are called PR3-ANCA and MPO-ANCA, respectively. MPO-ANCA is detected in 50–70 % of patients with MPA and 40–50 % of patients with CSS. PR3-ANCA is detected in 80–90 % of patients with GPA. Therapeutic apheresis is used in elderly patients with associated RPGN or pulmonary bleeding, who are at high risk for infections and are intolerant to standard immunosuppressive treatments.

26.5.2   Targets and Pathology

26.5.2.1   Targets

The targets of apheresis for AAV are autoantibodies (e.g., ANCA, anti-LAMP2 antibodies, antiplasminogen), activated leukocytes, activated macrophages, complement, adhesion molecules, cytokines, and chemokines.

26.5.2.2   Pathology

Environmental factors (infection, drugs etc.) in patients with susceptibility genes (e.g., *PTPN22, PDCD1, CTLA4*) trigger the activation of neutrophils, monocytes, and other immune cells, accelerating the secretion of inflammatory mediators such as TNFα and IL-1. MPO and PR3 are transported from primary cytoplasmic granules to the cell membrane during neutrophil activation and bind to ANCA. Binding of ANCA to endothelial cells increases adhesion molecule expression and cytokine production, resulting in damage to the endothelial cells of the vessel wall.

26.5.3   Efficacy

The efficacy of PE for MPA has been demonstrated in clinical trials. The MEPEX trial in MPA patients with severe renal dysfunction (serum creatinine >5.7 mg/dL) showed that the addition of PE versus intravenous methylprednisolone to oral cyclophosphamide and glucocorticoids was associated with a significantly better renal recovery rate at 3 and 12 months [18]. However, there was no difference in survival rate and renal survival rate between the two treatments [18]. Two subsequent meta-analyses, including the MEPEX trial, revealed that PE as adjunctive therapy significantly reduced the risk of endstage kidney disease at 12 months, but did not improve the survival rate [19, 20]. The ongoing multicenter PEXIVAS trial is evaluating the effectiveness of PE in patients with moderate renal failure (<50 mL/min estimated glomerular filtration rate).

An RCT was performed to evaluate the effectiveness of PE for patients with GPA, including those with moderately decreased renal function or renal failure [21]. The patients were randomized to treatment with or without initial PE in addition to oral cyclophosphamide and glucocorticoids; after 3 months they underwent a second randomization to continue cyclophosphamide or switch to cyclosporine A for 9 months. The renal survival rate and survival rate were significantly better in the PE group at 3 months. However, in the long-term follow-up of at least 5 years, the renal survival rate and survival rate were not significantly different. With regard to CSS, there have been no reports since the publication of a late 1990s study that failed to show the effectiveness of PE for CSS.

26.5.4   Methods

26.5.4.1   Insurance Restriction

Therapeutic apheresis is not approved for AAV.

26.5.4.2   Modality

(a) PE
(b) DFPP
(c) LCAP/GCAP

26.5.4.3   Frequency

PE is preferentially used for patients with AAV. It is initially performed two or three times a week. The treatment interval can be extended, according to the clinical response. DFPP is used for maintenance therapy.

26.5.4.4   Response Indicators

ANCA titers and CRP levels are used as indicators of response to therapy.

26.5.5   Points to Note

Refer to each section on apheresis.

References

1. Kempe K, Tsuda H, Yang K et al (2004) Filtration leukocytapheresis therapy in the treatment of rheumatoid arthritis patients resistant to or failed with methotrexate. Ther Apher Dial 8:197–205
2. Onuma S, Yamaji K, Kempe K et al (2006) Investigation of the clinical effect of large volume leukocytapheresis on methotrexate-resistant rheumatoid arthritis. Ther Apher Dial 10:404–411

3. Eguchi K, Saito K, Kondo M et al (2007) Enhanced effect of high-dose leukocytapheresis using a large filter in rheumatoid arthritis. Mod Rheumatol 17:481–485

4. Ueki Y, Sagawa A, Tanimura K et al (2007) A multicenter study of leuko-cytapheresis in rheumatoid arthritis. Clin Exp Rheumatol 25:810–816

5. Hiroshi Hashimoto; Kosei rodosho Kosei kagaku tokutei shikkan taisaku kenkyu jigyo nanchisei kekkanen ni kansuru chosa kenkyu han et al (2002) Nanchisei kekkanen no shinryo manyuaru Tokyo: [Kosei rodosho kosei kagaku tokutei shikkan taisaku kenkyu jigyo nanchisei kekkanen ni kansuru chosa kenkyu han] pp 35–40

6. Lewis EJ, Hunsicker LG, Lan SP et al (1992) A controlled trial of plasmapheresis therapy in severe lupus nephritis. The Lupus Nephritis Collaborative Study Group. N Engl J Med 326:1373–1379

7. Wallace DJ, Goldfinger D, Pepkowitz SH (1998) Randomized con-trolled trial of pulse/synchronization cyclophosphamide/apheresis for proliferative lupus nephritis. J Clin Apher 13:163–166

8. Danieli MG, Palmieri C, Salvi A et al (2002) Synchronised therapy and high-dose cyclophosphamide in proliferative lupus nephritis. J Clin Apher 17:72–77

9. Yamaji K, Kim YJ, Tsuda H et al (2002) Long-term clinical outcomes of synchronized therapy with plasmapheresis and intravenous cyclo-phosphamide pulse therapy in the treatment of steroid-resistant lupus nephritis. Ther Apher Dial 12:298–305

10. Loo CY, Mohamed Said MS, Mohd R et al (2010) Immunoadsorption and plasmapheresis are equally efficacious as adjunctive therapies for severe lupus nephritis. Transfus Apher Sci 43:335–340

11. Neuwelt CM (2003) The role of plasmapheresis in the treatment of severe central nervous system neuropsychiatric systemic lupus ery-thematosus. Ther Apher Dial 7:173–182

12. Hiroshi T (1993) Systemic lupus erythematosus In Japanese society for apheresis Plasmapheresis manual'93 Chugai-igakusha, Tokyo, pp186–190

13. Hickstein H, Külz T, Claus R, Stange J et al (2005) Autoimmune-associated congenital heart block: treatment of the mother with immunoadsorption. Ther Apher Dial 9:148–153

14. Miyakis S, Lockshin MD, Atsumi T et al (2006) International consen-sus statement on an update of the classification criteria for definite antiphospholipid syndrome (APS). J Thromb Haemost 4:295–306

15. Bucciarelli S, Espinosa G, Cervera R (2009) The CAPS Registry: morbidity and mortality of the catastrophic antiphospholipid syn-drome. Lupus 18:905–912

16. Ruffatti A, Marson P, Pengo V et al (2007) Plasma exchange in the management of high risk pregnant patients with primary antiphos-pholipid syndrome. A report of 9 cases and a review of the literature. Autoimmun Rev 6:196–202

17. Bortolati M, Marson P, Chiarelli S et al (2009) Case reports of the use of immunoadsorption or plasma exchange in high-risk

pregnancies of women with antiphospholipid syndrome. Ther Apher Dial 13:157–160

18. Jayne DR, Gaskin G, Rasmussen N et al (2007) Randomized trial of plasma exchange or high-dosage methylprednisolone as adjunctive therapy for severe renal vasculitis. J Am Soc Nephrol 18:2180–2188

19. Walters GD, Willis NS, Craig JC (2010) Interventions for renal vasculitis in adults. A systematic review. BMC Nephrol 11:12–35

20. Walsh M, Catapano F, Szpirt W et al (2011) Plasma exchange for renal vasculitis and idiopathic rapidly progressive glomerulonephritis: a meta-analysis. Am J Kidney Dis 57:566–574

21. Szpirt WM, Heaf JG, Petersen J (2011) Plasma exchange for induction and cyclosporine A for maintenance of remission in Wegener's granulomatosis – a clinical randomized controlled trial. Nephrol Dial Transplant 26:206–213

Chapter 27
Blood Type Incompatible Pregnancies

Norio Hanafusa

Main Points
- Antigens inherited from the father that the mother does not possess can be immunogenic when produced by the fetus, and antibodies can be produced in the maternal body against such antigens. Antibodies against paternal antigens on red blood cells can cause hemolytic anemia of the fetus.
- Fetal blood transfusion can be performed successfully in later gestation. However, during early gestation, until fetal blood transfusion can be performed safely, apheresis is applied.

27.1 Introduction

Blood type incompatible pregnancy can be observed in pregnancies where the mother does not have the antigen that the fetus has inherited from the father and she produces antibodies

N. Hanafusa (✉)
Department of Hemodialysis & Apheresis, University Hospital,
The University of Tokyo, 7-3-1 Hongo, Bunkyo-ku, Tokyo 113-8655, Japan
e-mail: hanafusa-tky@umin.ac.jp

E. Noiri and N. Hanafusa (eds.), *The Concise Manual
of Apheresis Therapy,* DOI 10.1007/978-4-431-54412-8_27,
© Springer Japan 2014

against the fetal antigen. IgG class antibodies can cross the placenta and cause hemolytic anemia within the fetus due to the antigen-antibody reaction. Fetal edema can be fatal.

Several blood types have been reported to cause blood type incompatible pregnancy. D antigen in the Rh system has the strongest antigenicity and can be clinically problematic. Prevention of sensitization through the use of immunoglobulin administration into the maternal body has been widely practiced and has led to a decreased prevalence of severe fetal anemia. Fetal blood transfusion has become a common practice to treat the hemolytic anemia observed in blood type incompatible pregnancies. Therefore, apheresis is rarely performed in this condition. However, during the period when fetal blood transfusion cannot be performed safely, which is until gestational week 18 or 19, apheresis is sometimes performed.

27.2 Target Conditions and Substances

27.2.1 Target Substances

Antibodies of IgG class (mainly anti-D antibody) against Rh blood group antigens are the main targets of apheresis.

27.2.2 Pathogenesis

Anti-D antibodies that are produced in the maternal body and enter into fetal circulation cause hemolytic anemia, which causes hepato-splenomegaly, or fetal edema.

Antibodies other than ones directed against P blood group antigens manifest mainly as hemolytic anemia. A transfusion of blood with the same blood type as the fetus or blood with O type, D(−), is performed after 18–19 weeks of gestation when such a transfusion into the fetus has become feasible. However, frequent fetal blood transfusions sometimes increases the titer of maternal anti-D antibodies.

Plasmapheresis is also often performed, especially in early gestation or in conditions where a rapid decrease in the antibody titer is required.

27.3   Actual Clinical Practice

27.3.1   Indication for Reimbursement

Treatment for blood type incompatible pregnancy can be reimbursed only for the presence of Rh blood group incompatibilities. The precise conditions include histories of intrauterine fetal distress or neonatal jaundice, and an indirect Coomb's test positive by more than 1:64 until gestation weeks 20, and by more than 1:128 for 20 weeks of gestation or later.

27.3.2   Modalities of Apheresis

Plasma exchange with 5 % albumin supplementation or double filtration plasmapheresis is chosen, because the aim of therapy is not supplementation of coagulation factors but antibody removal, and because there are some risks of infection due to unknown pathogens with use of FFP.

Heparin is used for anticoagulation, because the safety of nafamostat mesylate for fetuses remains unclear [1].

Dual lumen catheters should be avoided as much as possible, because the access has risks of sepsis. Therefore, a vascular access that is punctured before every session (i.e. direct puncture for central veins, superficial veins, or native brachial arteries) is preferred.

27.3.3   Treatment Frequency or Schedule

The rate is the same as ordinary plasmapheresis with 1–1.5 plasma volume (PV) of plasma exchanged. The frequency is modified between once to thrice a week according to the titer of the antibody. The process or exchange of 1–1.5 PV of plasma usually results in a reduction of the titer by one-half at the end of the session compared to that at the beginning (e.g. 1:1,024–1:512).

27.3.4   Clinical Indices

Until intrauterine fetal blood transfusions become available, it is recommended that the antibody titer should be kept at 1:512 or less [2].

The classification into zone one to three, according to bilirubin like substance in amniotic fluid (ΔOD450 value) and the gestational week, is used for an evaluation of the risks (Liley's chart or Queenan chart) [3]. Direct measurement of fetal hemoglobin or middle cerebral artery Doppler velocity has recently become available.

27.4   Points to Note

27.4.1   Fluctuation of Blood Pressure

Changes in oncotic pressure or electrolyte levels during plasmapheresis may cause a fluctuation of blood pressure that can affect placental blood flow. During the double filtration plasmapheresis (DFPP) procedure, changes in oncotic pressure change should be monitored with the use of a Crit-Line In-Line Monitor™ [In-Line Diagnostics, Kaysville, UT] (Fresenius Medical Care AG & Co. KGaA, Bad Homburg, Germany) The blood volume should not drop by more than 10 %. When blood volume changes greatly, the albumin infusion rate should be increased.

27.4.2   Bleeding Diathesis

Patients undergoing frequent plasmapheresis with albumin supplementation experience a reduction of those coagulation factors that possess longer half-lives such as fibrinogen or factor

XIII. The risks for perinatal bleeding increase when frequent apheresis is required until later gestation. The frequency of the therapies should be reduced, or coagulation factors can be supplemented, when fibrinogen, factor XIII, or immuno-globulin levels become profoundly decreased [1, 4]. On the other hand, hypercoagulation may occur during pregnancy and can be detected through thrombin-antithrombin complex measurement.

Note: Anti-PP$_1$P^k Antibody/Administration of Anti-D Immunoglobulin (RHIG) into Non-immunized Women/ Anti-phospholipid Antibody Syndrome

Anti-PP$_1$P^k antibody: P and P^k antigens found on the surface of erythrocytes are also expressed in the chorion. Anti-PP$_1$P^k antibodies found in the circulation of mothers without P, P$_1$, or P^k antigens (small p type) blood group antigens [1] can interfere with placental function, and result in intrauterine growth retardation or intra-uterine fetal loss. In such cases, apheresis therapy is suggested as early as possible; a patient who was treated as early as 5 weeks of gestation is reported. The apheresis treatment should be continued until late pregnancy, though the frequency can be reduced. However, blood type incompatible pregnancies, other than through the Rh system, are not reimbursed in Japan.

Administration of anti-D immunoglobulin (RHIG) into non-immunized women: Anti-D antibody injected intramuscularly can bind D-antigen positive blood cells derived from the fetus and prevent the production of anti-D antibodies. Blood cells of the fetus can be found in maternal circulation (feto-maternal transfusion). Therefore, when the mother does not have anti-D anti-bodies and the fetal blood type is D-positive, anti-D immunoglobulin is injected at 28 weeks of gestation and within 72 h after delivery. This strategy has been shown to profoundly decrease the incidence of seroconversion against D antigen from 13 % to 0.1 % [2].

> Anti-phospholipid antibody syndrome: Placental thrombus formation due to the presence of anti-phospholipid antibodies causes habitual abortion. Plasmapheresis has been reported to show efficacy to remove the antibody [5].

References

1. Hanafusa N et al (2006) Successful treatment by double filtrate plasmapheresis in a pregnant woman with the rare P blood group and a history of multiple early miscarriages. Ther Apher Dial 10(6):498–503
2. Omokawa S (2008) Blood purification therapy 2009: blood type incompatible pregnancy. Kidney Dial 65(Suppl):417–420 (in Japanese)
3. Sato A (2007) Diagnosis, therapy and management of obstetric disease: blood type incompatible pregnancy. J Jpn Obstet Gynecol Soc 59(12):N719–23 (in Japanese)
4. Hanafusa N et al (2007) Double filtration plasmapheresis can decrease factor XIII activity. Ther Apher Dial 11(3):165–70
5. Frampton G et al (1987) Successful removal of anti-phospholipid antibody during pregnancy using plasma exchange and low-dose prednisolone. Lancet 2(8566):1023–4

Chapter 28
Multiple Myeloma

Tsuyoshi Inoue

Main Points
- Plasma exchanges can be indicated when multiple myeloma or Waldenström's macroglobulinemia is diagnosed, but it is much more important to start the treatment of the underlying diseases themselves.
- Prompt plasma exchange should be considered when hyperviscosity syndrome is present.

28.1 Introduction

Renal failure is a major cause of morbidity and mortality in patients with multiple myeloma. Of those patients with newly diagnosed multiple myeloma, up to 50 % have renal impairment and 12–20 % have acute kidney injury, and among those patients with acute kidney injury, 10 % become dependent on dialysis. They represent 2 % of the dialysis population (0.4 % in Japan [1]) and there are approximately 5,000 new patients, worldwide, each year. The most common renal lesion is cast

---

T. Inoue (✉)
Division of Nephrology and Endocrinology, School of Medicine,
The University of Tokyo, 7-3-1 Hongo, Bunkyo-ku, Tokyo 113-8655, Japan
e-mail: tsinoue-tky@umin.ac.jp

E. Noiri and N. Hanafusa (eds.), *The Concise Manual of Apheresis Therapy,* DOI 10.1007/978-4-431-54412-8_28,
© Springer Japan 2014

nephropathy in the distal tubules, which leads to interstitial fibrosis. In these patients, a large amount of serum free light chains readily pass through the glomeruliand overwhelm the absorptive capacity of the proximal tubules [2].

Depending on the volume and types of M proteins, multiple myeloma can cause hyperviscosity syndrome. Waldenström's macroglobulinemia may also cause hyperviscosity syndrome, and when the symptoms are present, plasma exchange is indicated.

28.2   Multiple Myeloma

Multiple myeloma becomes increasingly common with age. Nowadays most people have regular medical checkups, and so it has become uncommon to see patients with myeloma who need urgent plasma exchange. While plasma exchanges have an immediate effect on multiple myeloma, it is mainly brought on by removing the offending proteins. Along with plasma exchange, it is necessary to start effective treatments that can significantly slow the production of light chains such as hematopoietic stem-cell transplantation with chemotherapy such as vincristine, doxorubicin, and dexamethasone (VAD) or melphalan and prednisolone (MP).

28.2.1   Therapeutic Targets (Objects and Medical Conditions)

28.2.1.1   Targeted Objects

Serum free light chains and M proteins are the targets of apheresis treatment in multiple myeloma.

28.2.1.2   Etiology

Removal of excess free light chains in the serum can be effective in patients who have acute renal failure with cast nephropathy. Plasma exchanges are indicated when cast nephropathy is proven by renal biopsy, and a large volume of light chains in serum or urine is confirmed. The standard schedule is five to six times for 7–10 days. There are some reports that hemodialysis or hemodiafiltration using a large pore dialyzer may be useful.

28.2.2   Effect of the Treatment

To date, three randomized clinical trials (RCTs) have been performed, and two of three showed the favorable effects of plasma exchange, but the latest and largest RCT of 97 patients showed no clinical meaningful difference [3]. The etiology of multiple myeloma is heterogenous and these studies have limitations. One small study was performed based on these results. That study suggested that when cast nephropathy can be confirmed, renal recovery seems to be highly associated with a significant reduction in serum levels of free light chains (over 50 % removal). This relationship was recently reported by others using a large pore dialyzer to remove pathologic light chains from patients with cast nephropathy [4].

In addition, it is reported that a large pore dialyzer can remove pathologic light chains from patients with cast nephropathy more efficiently than can plasma exchange [2, 5].

28.3   Hyperviscosity Syndrome

28.3.1   Therapeutic Targets (Objects and Medical Conditions)

28.3.1.1   Targeted Objects

Abnormal levels of IgA, IgG, and k-light chains in multiple myeloma can cause hyperviscosity. Compared to IgM, which forms 900 kDa-pentamer, the monomers of IgG, IgD, IgE, and the dimer of IgA are smaller. However, when the total number of immunoglobulin molecules increases, it can cause hyperviscosity syndrome. In addition, IgG3 and IgA can easily form high viscosity polymers that can lead to hyperviscosity syndrome.

28.3.1.2   Etiology

Hyperviscosity syndrome is triggered by an increase in serum proteins that can raise the viscosity of the plasma. Hyperviscosity leads to microcirculatory disturbances in the central nervous system, which can cause headache, vertigo, nystagmus, hearing impairment, visual disturbances, sleepiness, seizures, and coma. It can also cause heart failure and renal failure, and occasionally sausage-like dilation of the retinal veins caused by the expanded circulating plasma volume, as well as spontaneous bleeding from mucous membranes due to reduced platelet function.

28.3.2   Effect of the Treatment

The symptoms often rapidly improve with plasma exchange. After the cessation of treatment the symptoms often exacerbate, so it is important to treat the underlying disease itself as is the case with multiple myeloma treatment.

28.4   Therapeutic Protocol

28.4.1   Modality

Plasma exchange and double filtration plasmapheresis are the standard methods to remove pathogenetic plasma in patients. Cryofiltration is another treatment option, but basic plasma exchange is the simplest and most efficient. When the patients do not have impaired liver synthetic capacity or an abnormal hemostatic system, double filtration plasmapheresis can be applied and fresh frozen plasma (FFP) is not needed in such cases. The molecular weight of IgM is large, so it is necessary to use a large pore size membrane (such as EC-40W) as the secondary filter to remove IgM. As these kinds of membrane easily clog with IgM, frequent filter cleaning is needed.

Hemodialysis is sometimes required in patients with renal failure. FFP includes a large amount of acid citrate dextrose solution (ACD), which can lead to the dilution of proteins in FFP. When FFP is provided, a rapid drop of plasma oncotic pressure can occur and trigger severe complications such as pulmonary edema and brain edema. In addition, the sodium acid citrate in ACD may induce hypocalcemia and hypernatremia. Hemodialysis can remove water and sodium acid citrate, so it is safer to provide hemodialysis together with plasma exchange.

28.4.2   Treatment Schedule

The standard schedule is once weekly for 3 months. The rough standard volume of exchanging plasma per session is about 1–1.5 times the circulating plasma volume. When plasma exchange is indicated, the rapid removal of immunoglobulin such as IgG and IgM are required, so more frequent treatment is sometimes needed as noted earlier.

Because the circulating plasma volume is expanded due to the increase of plasma proteins in patients with hyperviscosity syndrome, the volume of exchanged plasma fluids may need to be increased.

28.4.3   Targeted Value

The goal of plasma exchange is to ameliorate acute renal failure or to reduce light chains in myeloma patients. In those patients with hyperviscosity syndrome, the goal is to improve the symptoms.

28.5   Safety Precaution

28.5.1   Hypotension

When the volume of M protein is large, the removal of M proteins with plasma exchange can cause hypotension due to the drop of colloid osmotic pressure. Equipment such as Crit-Line In-Line Monitor™ [In-Line Diagnostics, Kaysville, UT] should be used to monitor the change of blood volume. It is necessary to replenish albumin properly when the blood volume falls.

28.5.2   Bleeding Tendency

Patients with hyperviscosity syndrome may also have a bleeding tendency caused by abnormal platelet function. Patients with multiple myeloma may have a reduced number of platelets. When patients present with a bleeding tendency, nafamostat mesylate can be used as anticoagulant.

28.5.3   Precipitation of Cryoglobulin

Cryoglobulinemia may be encountered in patients with plasma cell dyscrasia such as multiple myeloma or Waldenström's macroglobulinemia. Cryoglobulins typically precipitate at temperatures below normal body temperature, so it is necessary to prevent the temperature in the circuit from becoming low enough to cause precipitation. This temperature differs among patients. However, cryofiltration, a procedure of plasmapheresis, selectively removes cryoprecipitates.

References

1. Nakai S et al (2012) Ther Apher Dial 16:11–53
2. Hutchinson CA et al (2007) J Am Soc Nephrol 18:886–895
3. Clark WF et al (2005) Ann Intern Med 143:777–784
4. Leung N et al (2008) Kidney Int 73:1282–1288
5. Hutchison CA et al (2009) Clin J Am Soc Nephrol 4:745–754

Chapter 29
Dilated Cardiomyopathy

Yoshifumi Hamasaki

> **Main Points**
> - Autoimmune disorders are considered to be one of the causes of dilated cardiomyopathy (DCM). Immunoglobulin G3 subclass antibodies are suggested to play a role in the pathogenesis of DCM.
> - Immunoadsorption plasmapheresis (IAPP) is a therapeutic apheresis treatment for DCM.
> - Because angiotensin converting enzyme inhibitor (ACE-I) drugs are contraindicated when IAPP with Imsorba® is performed, ACE-I therapy should be discontinued or switched to other drugs, such as an angiotensin II receptor blocker, before starting IAPP.

29.1   Introduction

Dilated cardiomyopathy (DCM) is an autoimmune-related cardiac disease for which apheresis treatment is indicated. DCM is defined as a group of diseases with cardiac dilatation

Y. Hamasaki (✉)
22nd Century Medical and Research Center, The University of Tokyo Hospital,
7-3-1 Hongo, Bunkyo-ku, Tokyo 113-8655, Japan
e-mail: yhamasaki-tky@umin.ac.jp

E. Noiri and N. Hanafusa (eds.), *The Concise Manual of Apheresis Therapy*, DOI 10.1007/978-4-431-54412-8_29,
© Springer Japan 2014

and severe contractile dysfunction. Patients with DCM can present with heart failure caused by contractile dysfunction, and can sometimes die suddenly from arrhythmia. Idiopathic DCM is diagnosed in the absence of the evident cause of cardiac dysfunction, such as coronary artery stenosis or secondary cardiomyopathy, as seen by coronary angiography or cardiac biopsy. The prevalence and total number of patients with idiopathic DCM in Japan, 14.0 per 100,000 population, and 17,700, respectively, were estimated in an epidemiological nationwide survey for patients undertook in 1999 [1].

Viral infections, familial (gene abnormality) causes, or autoimmune disorders are considered pathogenic factors for DCM. For those cases where autoimmune disorders are the cause, it is thought that DCM is caused by anti-myocardial antibodies (auto-antibodies against endogenous molecules such as $\beta 1$ adrenergic receptor, α-myosin heavy chain, β myosin heavy chain, M2 muscarinic receptor, troponin I, Na-K ATPase) [2, 3].

29.2   Pathogenesis of Dilated Cardiomyopathy and Target for Apheresis

29.2.1   Pathogenesis

Anti-myocardial antibodies play a role in the pathogenesis of DCM. Previous studies reported that serum anti-myocardial antibodies were detected in 38 % of symptomatic patients with DCM. It was demonstrated that the presence of anti-myocardial antibodies in the blood was related to the severity of heart failure and was predictive of mortality (all-cause mortality, cardiovascular mortality, and sudden death). Studies including showed that anti-myocardial antibodies were detected in 32 % of family members of patients with DCM, and that affected individuals also had a significantly higher occurrence rate of DCM [2]. These data suggest that anti-myocardial antibodies contribute to the onset and progress of DCM. It has been discovered recently that the treatment efficacy of immunoadsorption and IVIG is affected by polymorphism in the Fc gamma receptor IIa to which the Fc region of immunoglobulin G (IgG) binds [4].

29.2.2 Target of Apheresis

Because auto-antibodies contribute to the pathogenesis of DCM, the removal of IgG class antibodies has been tried as a treatment for DCM. In the IgG subclasses, IgG3 strongly binds complement components and can cause antibody-dependent cytotoxicity. In patients with DCM, a high titer of IgG3 subclass antibody is related to decreased left ventricular function. Because the IgG3 subclass has the strongest contribution to the pathogenesis of DCM among all IgG subclasses, IgG3 should be the main target of apheresis [2, 3].

29.3 Efficacy of Apheresis

A summary of the reports of apheresis treatment for DCM is shown in Table 29.1.

29.4 Method of Apheresis for DCM

29.4.1 Modality

Immunoadsorption plasmapheresis (IAPP) is a therapeutic apheresis for DCM [2, 3]. Plasma is isolated from whole blood of patients with DCM by a separation column, then the auto-antibodies (anti-myocardial antibodies) in the plasma are removed by the adsorption column. In 1996, Wallukat et al. first reported that the level of β1 adrenergic receptor antibodies in the serum of patients with DCM was decreased by IAPP [5].

Goat IgG antibody (Therasorb®), or protein A (Immunosorba®) which is a component of the cell wall of

TABLE 29.1 Previous reports of immunoadsorption for DCM

Year and journal	Authors	Number of patients	Ligand of adsorption column	Treatment duration	Results
1997, Circulation	Dorffel et al.	9	Sheep IgG	5 days	Hemodynamic status in acute phase was improved
2000, JACC	Felix et al.	9	Sheep IgG	4 courses	RCT. Hemodynamic status 3 months after treatment was improved
2004, Int J Cardiol	Dorffel et al.	9	Sheep IgG	4 courses	Follow up of above study for 3 years. Cardiac function was stable in persistent antibody-negative patients
2000, Circulation	Muller et al.	17	Sheep IgG	5 days	Symptom and hemodynamic status were improved
2004, Int J Cardiol	Knebel et al.	17	Sheep IgG	5 days	Follow up of above study for about 3 years. Hospital stay for heart failure was reduced
2002, JACC	Felix et al.	11	Sheep IgG	3 days	Hemodynamic status of early phase was improved
2002, Circulation	Staudt et al.	18	Protein A	4 courses	Removal of IgG3 was associated with improvement of hemodynamic status
2005, Am Heart J	Staudt et al.	18	Protein A	4 courses	Removal of IgG3 was associated with improvement of hemodynamic status

Year, Journal	Author	N	Column	Duration	Results
2006, Am Heart J	Staudt et al.	22	Protein A	1 course vs 6 courses	Improvement of cardiac function was not different between 2 groups after 6 months
2010, Am Heart J	Herda et al.	30	Protein A	5 days	Left ventricular function and ability to exercise were improved
2010, Eur J Clin Invest.	Trimpert et al.	17	Protein A	5 days	Myocardial antibody was not detected 6 months after treatment but elevated afterward
2010, J Clin Apher	Doesch et al.	51	Protein A	5 days	Left ventricular function and ability to exercise were improved after 6 months
2011, J Clin Apher	Nagatomo et al.	16	Tryptophan	3–5 times in 1–2 week(s)	Left ventricular function and ability to exercise were improved after 3 months

Staphylococcus aureus, is used as the ligand of the adsorption column. When adsorption columns with these ligands are used, it should be noted that immunoglobulin supplementation is needed and that the affinity for IgG3 of these ligands is weak. In Japan, Imsorba TR®, already used for IAPP treatment of myasthenia gravis or Guillain–Barré syndrome, is used as an adsorption column for IAPP treatment of DCM because of the following reasons: Imsorba TR® does not need Ig supplementation, it has a high specific affinity for IgG3 subclass among IgG classes, and it is safe because the adsorbent of Imsorba TR® is made from tryptophan [2].

29.4.2 Frequency

Along with an increase in treated plasma volume, serum bradykinin level is elevated and the removal of fibrinogen from IAPP causes coagulation abnormalities. Considering these adverse effects, in addition to the efficacy for IgG of Imsorba TR®, the amount of plasma volume to be treated with IAPP with Imsorba TR® has been determined to be 1,500 mL per session. IAPP treatment is performed for around 2 h per session with less than 100 mL/min blood flow and less than 20 mL/min plasma flow. A clinical trial of IAPP with Imsorba TR® for DCM is now being conducted in Japan with the following protocol: IAPP with Imsorba TR® with a treated plasma volume of 1,500 mL per session performed every other day (three times per week) and five times in total, which is then repeated once more.

29.4.3 Target Markers

Target markers are an improvement of cardiac function (cardiac ultrasonography, Swan–Ganz catheter examination) and the ability to exercise, and humoral markers (BNP, NT-Pro BNP). Measurements of titers for myocardial antibodies are also performed.

29.4.4   Precaution for Treatment

Bradykinin production is increased when the kallikrein–kinin system is enhanced by the negatively charged Imsorba TR®. Angiotensin converting enzyme inhibitor (ACE-I) adminis-tration accelerates the accumulation of bradykinin in the body by inhibiting its metabolism. This increased level of bradykinin could trigger shock or hypotension. Therefore, when IAPP with Imsorba TR® is performed, the use of ACE-I is contraindicated. Before starting IAPP, therapy with ACE-I should be discontinued or switched to another drug such as an angiotensin II receptor blocker.

References

1. Miura K et al (2002) Epidemiology of idiopathic cardiomyopathy in Japan: results from a nationwide survey. Heart 87(2):126–130
2. Yoshikawa T et al (2009) Autoimmune mechanisms underlying dilated cardiomyopathy. Circ J 73:602–607
3. Felix SB et al (2008) Immunoadsorption as treatment option in dilated cardiomyopathy. Autoimmunity 41(6):484–489
4. Staudt A et al (2010) Fc gamma-receptor IIa polymorphism and the role of immunoadsorption in cardiac dysfunction in patients with dilated cardiomyopathy. Clin Pharmacol Ther 87(4):452–458
5. Wallukat G et al (1996) Removal of autoantibodies in dilated cardiomyopathy by immunoadsorption. Int J Cardiol 54(2):191–195

Part V
Pathogens with Large Molecular Weight

Chapter 30
Low Density Lipoprotein Apheresis

Kenjiro Honda and Kent Doi

Main Points

- Therapeutic plasma exchange volume is usually 3–5 L/session.
- Removal of positively charged particles as well as low density lipoprotein cholesterol improves focal segmental glomerulosclerosis and peripheral arterial disease.
- Angiotensin converting enzyme (ACE) inhibitors should be discontinued at least 2–3 days prior to low density lipoprotein (LDL) apheresis.
- LDL apheresis should be performed with careful attention to its promotion of bleeding tendencies because of the adsorption of endogenous coagulation factors.

K. Honda (✉)
Department of Nephrology and Endocrinology, University Hospital,
The University of Tokyo, 7-3-1 Hongo, Bunkyo-ku, Tokyo 113-8655, Japan
e-mail: khonda-tky@umin.ac.jp

K. Doi
Department of Emergency and Critical Care Medicine, University Hospital,
The University of Tokyo, 7-3-1 Hongo, Bunkyo-ku, Tokyo 113-8655, Japan

E. Noiri and N. Hanafusa (eds.), *The Concise Manual of Apheresis Therapy*, DOI 10.1007/978-4-431-54412-8_30, © Springer Japan 2014

30.1   Introduction

Low density lipoprotein (LDL), with a specific gravity of
1.019–1.063 g/mL and a particle size of 19–22 nm, is recognized as a causative molecule of atherosclerosis. Foam cells,
formed by macrophages that accumulate modified LDL
cholesterol, like oxidized LDL cholesterol, promote atherosclerosis. In addition, hyperlipidemia is a risk factor for
myocardial infarction.

LDL apheresis is a therapeutic modality to eliminate LDL
cholesterol from the bloodstream through extracorporeal
circulation. The Liposorber system (Kaneka) uses a ligand of
dextran sulfate. Because the dextran sulfate group is negatively charged, it electrostatically binds to positively charged
particles. Therefore, the system adsorbs molecules such as
very low density lipoprotein (VLDL) cholesterol that includes
apoB lipoproteins.

30.2   Indication for LDL Apheresis

The first clinical report for LDL apheresis detailed two cases
of familial hypercholesterolemia in 1975 [1]. At present,
apheresis is applicable for familial hypercholesterolemia
(FH), lower limb peripheral arterial disease, and focal segmental glomerulosclerosis. Indication criteria are described
in Table 30.1.

30.2.1   Familial Hypercholesterolemia

FH typically is manifest through autosomal dominant inheri-
tance, predominantly with LDL receptor gene disorder. In
FH patients, a prolonged half-life of LDL cholesterol results
in hypercholesterolemia. Heterozygous FH occurs in 1:500
while homozygous FH in 1:10,000, and LDL cholesterol
clearance in these two forms is decreased by 53 % and 27 %,
respectively. Progression of atherosclerosis, even in younger

TABLE 30.1 Indications for LDL apheresis

Disease	Indication criteria
Familial hypercholesterolemia (FH)	• Persistent cases with hypercholesterolemia (total cholesterol ≥ 220 mg/dL or LDL cholesterol ≥ 140 mg/dL) refractory to drug administration
Peripheral arterial disease (PAD) of lower extremities	Cases that fulfill the following criteria • Symptomatic cases that are more severe than or equal to Fontaine classification II • Persistent hypercholesterolemia (total cholesterol ≤ 220 mg/dL or LDL cholesterol ≤ 140 mg/dL) refractory to drug administration • Patients refractory to conventional medication treatment without an indication for surgical therapy due to distal lesions below the knee or diffuse lesions
Focal segmental glomerulosclerosis (FSGS)	• Nephrotic syndrome resistant to corticosteroid therapy with total cholesterol more than 250 mg/dL

ages, leads to the development of coronary artery disease and short life expectancy. The genetic mutation of the LDL receptor is classified into the following four types based on the variance of the protein [2].

Class 1: The LDL receptor protein is not synthesized.

Class 2: Despite normal synthesis of LDL receptor protein in the endoplasmic reticulum, an inhibition of transport from the endoplasmic reticulum to Golgi body prevents the receptor expression on the cell surface.

Class 3: Although receptor protein expression is normal, an LDL receptor abnormality makes it impossible to bind LDL.

Class 4: Despite normal binding to the LDL receptor, a disorder of transport to coated pits inhibits intracellular LDL transport.

LDL cholesterol accumulation in the skin, tendons, and arterial walls causes xanthoma, tendon thickening, and atheroma formation. In addition, aortic valve stenosis occurs due to atherosclerosis of the aortic arch in approximately half of homozygous cases.

30.2.2 Lower Limb Peripheral Arterial Disease

Arteriosclerosis obliterans (ASO) is now considered to be a part of peripheral arterial disease (PAD) whose lesion area extends beyond the lower extremities. The number of patients with PAD is increasing, and is now estimated to be four million. Arteries in the lower extremities are a frequent site in PAD, and Fontaine's classification is used to assess the severity (Table 30.2). In patients with chronic symptoms of numbness and intermittent claudication, neuropathy caused by lumbar canal stenosis is considered in the differential diagnosis. Stenotic lesions are often presumed by symptomatic sites in intermittent claudication. PAD progression leads to a shortening of the claudication distance and the appearance of rest pain or intractable ulcers. The rest pain is frequently noticed during nighttime, while it is relieved by a seated position or knee flexion. Advanced PAD, such as critical limb ischemia (CLI), with intractable ulcers or gangrene, occasionally requires opioids for intolerable pain. Patients with CLI have insomnia and delirium with pain, and severe infection with methicillin resistant *Staphylococcus aureus* or *Pseudomonas aeruginosa*. Chronic inflammation with ulcers or gangrene also induces appetite loss and malnutrition.

Treatment for PAD of the lower extremities in an early phase includes exercise, medication management using antiplatelet or peripheral vasodilator drugs, and management for atherosclerosis risk factors such as chronic kidney disease, diabetes mellitus and dyslipidemia. Revascularization including percutaneous transluminal angioplasty (PTA) and bypass surgery should be taken into consideration in cases with rapid progression. However, revascularization is difficult to

TABLE 30.2 Severity categories in lower limb peripheral arterial disease

Fontaine classification		Rutherford classification	
Stage	**Clinical symptoms**	**Stage**	**Clinical symptoms**
1	No symptoms	0	Asymptomatic
2a	Intermittent claudication without pain on resting, but with claudication at a distance of greater than 650 feet (200 m)	1	Mild claudication
2b	Intermittent claudication without pain on resting, but with a claudication distance of less than 650 feet (200 m)	2	Moderate claudication
		3	Severe claudication
3	Nocturnal and/or resting pain	4	Rest pain
4	Necrosis (death of tissue) and/or gangrene in the limb	5	Ischemic ulceration not exceeding ulcer of the digits of the foot
		6	Severe ischemic ulcers or frank gangrene

perform in patients with diffuse lesions or distal lesions under the knee. CLI treatment includes LDL apheresis, hyperbaric therapy, blood stem cell transplantation, and maggot debridement therapy, as well as revascularization for those with poor prognosis or difficult-to-treat cases. Immediately after beginning LDL apheresis, patients will occasionally experience some relief of ischemic symptoms, and LDL apheresis has been reported to promote collateral vessel formation in angiographic findings.

Although serum cholesterol values return to baseline level within 2 weeks after the end of LDL apheresis, the improvement of symptoms continues in some cases. LDL apheresis also has been reported to ameliorate SPP and ABI, improve distance to claudication, and reduce pain level, and area of ulcers [3]. Table 30.3 shows the mechanisms of the effect of LDL apheresis on PAD, including vasodilatation caused by an increased production of nitric oxide and bradykinin, a

TABLE 30.3 Therapeutic mechanism of LDL apheresis in lower limb peripheral arterial disease

Effect on blood or plasma	Improvement of erythrocyte deformability, lowering of plasma viscosity, improvement of microcirculation by adsorption of coagulation factors
Vasodilatation	Production of nitric oxide, bradykinin, and prostaglandin I_2, reduction of endothelin-1
Angiogenesis	Production of vascular growth factors (HGF, VEGF), increasing collateral vessel formation
Protection from atherosclerotic progression	Anti-inflammatory action including the inhibition of cytokine expression and decreasing levels of C-reactive protein, P-selectin (platelet adhesion factor), and monocyte migration factor (MCP-1), improvement of vascular endothelial function, lipid lowering effect

Adapted from information in [4–7]

reduction of blood viscosity, and an improvement of rheology [4–7]. Furthermore, angiogenesis and the suppression of adhesion molecule expression among blood cells induced by cytokines such as vascular endothelial growth factor (VEGF) have been reported. It is expected that a novel mechanism for the improvements seen with the therapy will be discovered.

30.2.3   Focal Segmental Glomerulosclerosis

Focal segmental glomerulosclerosis (FSGS) has pathological features consisting of a focal distribution of sclerotic lesions in glomeruli. Although the concise mechanism of the development remains unclear, the cause is considered to include the disorder of factors that regulate permeability in glomeruli and genetic factors of susceptibility to podocyte injury [8]. FSGS tends to develop refractory nephrotic syndrome and have a poor renal prognosis. The peak age of onset is relatively young, and patients older than 50 years are rare. A renal biopsy is necessary for definite diagnosis, and light microscopy will show that some glomeruli are normal and that the others have segmental sclerotic lesions. An immunofluorescence study will usually show IgM and C3 deposition in the sclerotic segment. However, in some cases, it is difficult to differentiate FSGS with minimal change nephrotic syndrome. The clinical findings in FSGS are poor corticosteroid responsiveness, red blood cell casts and granular casts in urinary sediment, low urinary selectivity index, and podocyte desquamation in urine. Persistent and marked hypercholesterolemia is considered to exasperate glomerular sclerosis and deteriorate kidney function. LDL apheresis is reported to be effective for improving remission rates of FSGS via remedying hypercholesterolemia and inflammation. Because hypercholesterolemia is thought to inhibit the effect of some drugs, LDL apheresis is a notable therapy in that it improves the effect of corticosteroid and cyclosporine.

30.3   Devices and Methods of LDL Apheresis

Several devices are available in LDL apheresis (see Table 30.4). In both Liposorber systems (Kaneka) and double filtration plasmapheresis (DFPP) systems, the primary membrane performs plasma separation followed by an adsorption column or secondary membrane. LDL cholesterol is eliminated by adsorption or molecular sieving, but the removal rates are similar between the two systems.

Examples of therapeutic plans are twice a week for 6 weeks (for 5 weeks in PAD) or twice a week for 6 weeks followed by once a week for 6 weeks. Blood flow rate and plasma flow rate are 50–100 mL/min and 15–30 mL/min, respectively. The objective for total plasma volume treated is 3–5 L/session.

TABLE 30.4 Devices of LDL apheresis

	Liposorber	DFPP	AS-15, AS-25
Manufacturer	Kaneka	Asahi Kasei Kuraray Medical	Kaneka
Perfusion system	Plasma perfusion	Plasma perfusion	Direct blood perfusion
Plasma separator	Plasmaflo OP	Plasmaflo OP	Unnecessary
Secondary membrane	None	Cascadeflo EC	Unnecessary
Adsorbent	LA-15 500 mL LA-40S 400 mL	None	AS-15 150 mL AS-25 250 mL
Carrier	Cellulose beads	None	cellulose beads
Ligand	Dextran sulfate	None	Dextran sulfate, tryptophan
Action	Electrostatic interaction	Sieving	Electrostatic interaction Hydrophobic interaction
LDL removal	50–70 %	50–70 %	20 %
Bradykinin production	+	–	+
System	Complicated	Moderate	Easy
Indication	FH, PAD, FSGS	PAD	PAD

Adapted from information in [3]

30.4   Treatment Precaution

30.4.1   Withdrawal of ACE Inhibitors

In LDL apheresis using Liposorber LA-15, the negatively charged dextran sulfate column activates intrinsic clotting factors. This induces bradykinin with the vasodilator effect, whereas angiotensin-converting enzyme (ACE) inhibitors inhibit bradykinin metabolism. Because an anaphylactoid reaction during LDL apheresis has been described in patients taking ACE inhibitors, ACE inhibitor administration should be discontinued at least 2–3 days prior to the treatment. This phenomenon is avoidable when nafamostat mesylate is used as an anticoagulant because it suppresses bradykinin production through the inhibition of kallikrein.

30.4.2   Hypotension

In patients with atherosclerosis progression, a reduction of vascular compliance, or the presence of ischemic heart disease, LDL apheresis frequently brings about a reduction in blood pressure. For those patients with the possibility of blood pressure reduction during treatment, it is recommended that the blood flow is started with a low flow rate, or that an albumin prime is performed (See Chap. 17).

30.4.3   Bleeding Tendency

LDL apheresis may promote bleeding tendency through the adsorption of coagulation factors. Treatment requires considerable attention to bleeding complications because antiplatelet drugs or prostaglandin analogues are frequently prescribed for cardiovascular comorbidities. Precautions to take are screening for gastrointestinal bleeding before LDL apheresis, monitoring fibrinogen levels during the duration of treatment, and assessing the necessity of lowering the dose of antiplatelet drugs or prostaglandin analogues (See Chap. 18).

Note: Enlargement of Indications for LDL Apheresis
Japanese medical insurance covers FH, PAD, and FSGS as indications for LDL apheresis in 2010. However, some reports have shown the effectiveness of LDL apheresis for other diseases, including diabetic nephropathy, where it can cause a decrease of serum creatinine and proteinuria [9], and for FH patients after ischemic heart disease, where it can improve reperfusion to the myocardium and can help prevent coronary restenosis [10]. LDL apheresis is also considered to be effective in PAD patients with low cholesterol levels who receive regular dialysis, based on mechanisms other than simply reducing serum cholesterol. Taking these points into consideration, an enlargement of the indications for LDL apheresis should be considered.

References

1. Thompson GR, Lowenthal R, Myant NB (1975) Plasma exchange in the management of homozygous familial hypercholesterolaemia. Lancet 1:1208–11
2. Hobbs HH, Russell DW, Brown MS et al (1990) The LDL receptor locus in familial hypercholesterolemia: mutational analysis of a membrane protein. Annu Rev Genet 24:133–70
3. Ohtake T, Kobayashi S (2009) Masshodoumyakushikkan nitaisuru atarashii chokusetsukanryuu (DHP) chiryo. Jpn J Apher 28:224–9
4. Kobayashi S, Moriya H, Negishi K et al (2003) LDL-apheresis up-regulates VEGF and IGF-I in patients with ischemic limb. J Clin Apher 18:115–9
5. Kobayashi S, Moriya H, Maesato K et al (2005) LDL-apheresis improves peripheral arterial occlusive disease with an implication for anti-inflammatory effects. J Clin Apher 20:239–43
6. Kobayashi S, Oka M, Moriya H et al (2006) LDL-apheresis reduces P-Selectin, CRP and fibrinogen – possible important implications for improving atherosclerosis. Ther Apher Dial 10:219–23
7. Kobayashi S (2008) Applications of LDL-apheresis in nephrology. Clin Exp Nephrol 12:9–15
8. Mitarai T (2002) Sojoshikyutaikokasho. Sogorinsho 81:547–52

9. Kobayashi S (1998) LDL-Apheresis for diabetic nephropathy: a possible new tool. Nephron 79:505–6
10. Aengevaeren WR, Kroon AA, Stalenhoef AF et al (1996) Low density lipoprotein apheresis improves regional myocardial perfusion in patients with hypercholesterolemia and extensive coronary artery disease. LDL-Apheresis Atherosclerosis Regression Study (LAARS). J Am Coll Cardiol 28:1696–704

Chapter 31
Endotoxin Absorption Therapy

Kent Doi

> **Main Points**
> - Endotoxin (lipopolysaccharide, LPS), a component of the gram-negative bacterial cell wall, is recognized as the most potent microbial mediator implicated in the pathogenesis of sepsis.
> - Removal of circulating endotoxin by hemoperfusion through an immobilized polymyxin B (PMX-B) column (direct hemoperfusion with PMX-B column; PMX-DHP) reportedly improves outcomes in cases of sepsis [1].

31.1 Role of Endotoxin in Sepsis

Sepsis is recognized as the systemic host response to invasive infection, in which hyper-immunological reactions highlighted by elevated blood cytokine levels occur. Sepsis is

K. Doi(✉)
Department of Emergency and Critical Care Medicine, University Hospital, The University of Tokyo, 7-3-1 Hongo, Bunkyo-ku, Tokyo 113-8655, Japan
e-mail: kdoi-tky@umin.ac.jp

E. Noiri and N. Hanafusa (eds.), *The Concise Manual of Apheresis Therapy,* DOI 10.1007/978-4-431-54412-8_31,
© Springer Japan 2014

326   K. Doi

Table 31.1 Definition of SIRS

	Parameters
Temperature	<36 °C (96.8 °F) or >38 °C (100.4 °F)
Heart rate	>90 beats per minute
Respiratory rate	>20 per minute or $PaCO_2$ <32 mm Hg
WBC	<4,000/mm^3, >12,000/mm^3, or 10 % band

Systemic inflammatory response syndrome (SIRS) can be diagnosed when two or more of these criteria are present

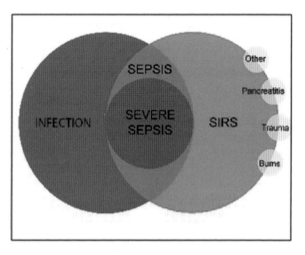

Figure 31.1 The relationship between systematic inflammatory response syndrome (SIRS), infection, and sepsis

clinically defined as systemic inflammatory response syndrome (SIRS) caused by infection (Table 31.1 and Fig. 31.1) [2]. Endotoxin (lipopolysaccharide; LPS) plays a crucial role in triggering the overreaction of the immunological defense system. In addition, sepsis induces changes of systemic hemodynamics that evolve from an early hyperdynamic ("warm shock") state to a late hypodynamic ("cold shock") state. Similar hemodynamic changes were reportedly observed after a large LPS injection [3]. This supports the view that it is not the bacterial infection itself, but rather the LPS that directly contributes to the pathophysiology of septic shock.

31.2   Removal of Endotoxin

It has been demonstrated that the polymyxin B (PMX-B) molecule has both antibacterial and anti-endotoxin capabilities. PMX-B can bind to lipid A located in the active center of the LPS and neutralize the activity. An extracorporeal device (Toraymyxin PMX-F; Toray, Tokyo, Japan), where the PMX-B is grafted on sorbent material and is able to provide selective removal of circulating endotoxin, is clinically available in several countries in Europe and Asia. The use of this extracorporeal cartridge avoids the side effects of systemic administration of PMX-B such as nephrotoxicity and neurotoxicity.

Although immobilized PMX-B column therapy appears to be effective only in gram-negative bacterial infections, it might have protective effects against gram-positive bacterial infections. Reportedly, PMX-B columns adsorb not only LPS but also anandamide, and they inhibit the cytotoxic effect of endogenous cannabinoid [4]. Because cannabinoids are known to have hypotensive effects, the vasopressor action by the PMX-B column may be at least partly derived from adsorption of the endogenous cannabinoid.

31.3   Effects of PMX Direct Hemoperfusion on Sepsis

A meta-analysis evaluating 28 clinical studies on endotoxin adsorption therapy reported clinical improvements on mean blood pressure, oxygenation, and survival rate, and the requirement for presser medications [1]. A multicenter randomized control trial on the effects of PMX direct hemoperfusion (DHP) on sepsis was conducted recently (EUPHAS study) [5]. Sixty-four patients who had undergone abdominal surgery complicated with severe sepsis or septic shock were randomly assigned into the PMX-DHP group and the conventional treatment group. In the PMX-DHP group, significantly higher mean blood pressures and fewer amounts of required presser medications were observed. The PMX-DHP group showed a better 28 day mortality rate, although the 60 day mortality rate did not show any significant difference between the groups [6]. Two multicenter randomized control trials on PMX-DHP are now underway, one in the US (EUPHRATES study) and one in Europe (ABDO-MIX study).

31.4   Procedures of PMX Direct Hemoperfusion

31.4.1   Limitation of Insurance System in Japan

In Japan, PMX-DHP is indicated for severely ill patients (SIRS as shown in Table 31.1) with endotoxemia or gram-negative bacterial infection. The endotoxin activity assay (EAA) has recently been approved by the US FDA as an ex-vivo diagnostic test of endotoxemia. It requires only 30 min to measure blood endotoxin levels as endotoxin activity (EA) values that are expressed in relative units derived from the integral of the basal and maximally stimulated chemiluminescent responses [7]. The Multi-Center Endotoxin Detection in Critical Illness (MEDIC) study demonstrated that higher EA levels are associated with a higher risk of mortality, as well as an increased risk for developing sepsis [8].

31.4.2   Columns for PMX Direct Hemoperfusion

Two different sizes of PMX-B immobilized columns are clinically available (Toraymyxin PMX-F, Toray, Tokyo, Japan) (Table 31.2). PMX-20R columns can remove a total amount of 1.1 mg endotoxin. The smaller column (PMX-05R) is used not only in pediatrics but also for very aged patients or underweight patients (<40 kg) [9].

TABLE 31.2 PMX-B immobilized column

	PMX-20R	PMX-05R
Length	225 mm	133 mm
Diameter	63 mm	55 mm
Weight	56 ± 3 g	15 ± 2 g
Blood volume	135 ± 3 mL	40 ± 3 mL
Blood flow	80–120 mL/min	20–40 mL/min

PMX-B polymyxin B

31.4.3   Timing and Schedule of PMX Direct Hemoperfusion

Under the Japanese insurance system, two consecutive sessions of PMX-DHP every 24 h are usually provided. Treatment time is described as 2 h on the product label, however, PMX-B immobilized columns appear to be able to remove endotoxin for more than 2 h. Some Japanese physicians prefer to perform PMX-DHP for as long as 6 h. Further evaluation is necessary to confirm the optimal treatment time.

It is important to conduct PMX-DHP when the source of endotoxin is under control, e.g., surgical drainage has been completed or is under consideration. Otherwise, a rebound of blood endotoxin levels will cause a second episode of septic shock. Early initiation of treatment at warm shock status will improve patients' outcomes compared with starting at the cold shock stage or when there is multiple organ failure, although no clinical study has evaluated the optimal starting time of PMX-DHP.

31.5   Complications

31.5.1   Thrombocytopenia

Not only endotoxin but also platelets are absorbed by PMX-B immobilized columns. Observation by electronic microscopy will show platelet pseudopodia, which indicates platelet activation. The impact of PMX-DHP on platelet count depends on the absolute platelet counts in the blood. For instance, PMX-DHP will reduce platelet counts from 150,000–200,000/mL to 100,000/mL, however, it will not reduce the values when pre-PMX-DHP platelet counts are approximately 50,000/mL.

Note: PMX-DHP May Have Other Effects Beyond Endotoxin Absorption

1. PMX-DHP may improve acute interstitial pneumonitis (AIP), acute exacerbation of idiopathic interstitial pneumonia, or acute lung injury/adult respiratory distress syndrome (ALI/ARDS). A single center clinical study reported PMX-DHP improved oxygenation and reduced inflammatory cytokines of KL-6 in respiratory failure patients whose blood endotoxin levels were below the detectable limit [10].Possible mechanisms of lung protection by PMX-DHP are considered to be the suppression of activated neutrophils and the reduction of levels of inflammatory cytokines [11].

2. Inflammation in sepsis is largely initiated by toll-like receptors (TLRs), which detect not only a wide range of microbial diversity, but also cellular constituents released due to tissue injury, triggering innate immune responses. Myeloid differentiation factor 88 (MyD88) is an adaptor protein for all TLRs, except TLR3, linking receptors with downstream kinases. These MyD88-dependent pathways induce the activation of nuclear factor κB (NF-κB) and cytokine production such as tumor necrosis factor α (TNF-α). TLR4 recognizes LPS, whereas TLR2 binds to the lipoprotein of gram-positive bacteria cell walls and the TLR9 signal is induced by CpG DNA derived from bacteria. All these signals seem to induce MyD88-mediated signals and enhance

inflammatory reactions in sepsis. Therefore, the removal of endotoxin alone, which may reduce TLR4-dependent reactions, will not sufficiently improve sepsis. Considering the effects of PMX-DHP on gram-positive infections and pulmonary diseases, PMX-DHP may work in several different pathways in addition to endotoxin removal. Further research is necessary to clarify this hypothesis.

References

1. Cruz DN, Perazella MA, Bellomo R, de Cal M, Polanco N, Corradi V, Lentini P, Nalesso F, Ueno T, Ranieri VM, Ronco C (2007) Effectiveness of polymyxin B-immobilized fiber column in sepsis: a systematic review. Crit Care 11:R47
2. Bone RC, Balk RA, Cerra FB, Dellinger RP, Fein AM, Knaus WA, Schein RM, Sibbald WJ (1992) American College of Chest Physicians/ Society of Critical Care Medicine Consensus Conference: definitions for sepsis and organ failure and guidelines for the use of innovative therapies in sepsis. Crit Care Med 20:864–874
3. Taveira da Silva AM, Kaulbach HC, Chuidian FS, Lambert DR, Suffredini AF, Danner RL (1993) Brief report: shock and multiple-organ dysfunction after self-administration of Salmonella endotoxin. N Engl J Med 328:1457–1460
4. Wang Y, Liu Y, Sarker KP, Nakashima M, Serizawa T, Kishida A, Akashi M, Nakata M, Kitajima I, Maruyama I (2000) Polymyxin B binds to anandamide and inhibits its cytotoxic effect. FEBS Lett 470:151–155
5. Cruz DN, Antonelli M, Fumagalli R, Foltran F, Brienza N, Donati A, Malcangi V, Petrini F, Volta G, Bobbio Pallavicini FM, Rottoli F, Giunta F, Ronco C (2009) Early use of polymyxin B hemoperfusion in abdominal septic shock: the EUPHAS randomized controlled trial. JAMA 301:2445–2452
6. Kida Y (2009) Polymyxin B hemoperfusion and mortality in abdominal septic shock. JAMA 302:1969 (Author reply 1969–1970)
7. Romaschin AD, Harris DM, Ribeiro MB, Paice J, Foster DM, Walker PM, Marshall JC (1998) A rapid assay of endotoxin in whole blood using autologous neutrophil dependent chemiluminescence. J Immunol Methods 212:169–185

8. Marshall JC, Foster D, Vincent JL, Cook DJ, Cohen J, Dellinger RP, Opal S, Abraham E, Brett SJ, Smith T, Mehta S, Derzko A, Romaschin A (2004) Diagnostic and prognostic implications of endotoxemia in critical illness: results of the MEDIC study. J Infect Dis 190:527–534

9. Nakamura T, Kawagoe Y, Ueda Y, Koide H (2005) Polymyxin B-immobilized fiber hemoperfusion with low priming volume in an elderly septic shock patient with marked endotoxemia. ASAIO J 51:482–484

10. Seo Y, Abe S, Kurahara M, Okada D, Saito Y, Usuki J, Azuma A, Koizumi K, Kudoh S (2006) Beneficial effect of polymyxin B-immobilized fiber column (PMX) hemoperfusion treatment on acute exacerbation of idiopathic pulmonary fibrosis. Intern Med 45:1033–1038

11. Kushi H, Miki T, Okamaoto K, Nakahara J, Saito T, Tanjoh K (2005) Early hemoperfusion with an immobilized polymyxin B fiber column eliminates humoral mediators and improves pulmonary oxygenation. Crit Care 9:R653–R661

Part VI
Diseases Necessary to Supply Coagulation Factors

Chapter 32
Liver Disease

Kent Doi

> **Main Points**
> - Apheresis is one of the possible therapeutic strategies for acute liver failure, such as that caused by fulminant hepatitis and post-surgery liver failure.
> - Plasma exchange (PE) plays an important role as an artificial liver support (ALS) until progressive hepatocyte necrosis ends and sufficient hepatic regeneration occurs.
> - Liver transplantation has recently improved the prognosis of fulminant hepatitis. Preoperative conditions, especially hepatic coma, are known to have a great impact on the survival rates associated with liver transplantation. Therefore, apheresis in fluminant hepatitis is necessary as a bridge therapy to transplantation.

K. Doi (✉)
Department of Emergency and Critical Care Medicine, University Hospital,
The University of Tokyo, 7-3-1 Hongo, Bunkyo-ku, Tokyo 113-8655, Japan
e-mail: kdoi-tky@umin.ac.jp

E. Noiri and N. Hanafusa (eds.), *The Concise Manual*
of Apheresis Therapy, DOI 10.1007/978-4-431-54412-8_32,
© Springer Japan 2014

335

32.1   Liver Diseases Treated by Apheresis

32.1.1   Fulminant Hepatitis

Fulminant hepatitis usually presents as severe acute liver failure complicated with bleeding tendency and hepatic coma. The Japanese definition of fulminant hepatitis is shown in Table 32.1; the subacute type shows a worse prognosis. The causes of fulminant hepatitis include viral infections and drug and autoimmune reactions (Table 32.2). However, the subacute type frequently has no clear cause. Yoshiba and colleagues have developed an original algorithm that can predict fulminant hepatitis. They reported the importance of prediction of fluminant hepatitis by this algorithm in acute hepatitis without any hepatic coma but with prothrombin time <40 % (Table 32.3) [1].

TABLE 32.1 Diagnosis of fulminant hepatitis

Fulminant hepatitis is defined when the following two criteria are met: (1) hepatic coma (grade II) within 8 weeks after the onset and (2) prothrombin time below 40 %

Acute type: coma occurs within 10 days of onset

Subacute type: coma occurs 11 days or later after onset

TABLE 32.2 Causes of fulminant hepatitis

	Acute	Subacute
Hepatitis B virus	64.7 %	28.7 %
Hepatitis A virus	3.3 %	0.0 %
Drug reaction	11.7 %	18.5 %
Unknown	20.8 %	52.8 %

Data from national survey of Japan in 2003–2005 [3]

TABLE 32.3 Prediction score for fulminant hepatitis

$Z = -0.89 + 1.74 \times$ viral infection ($1 =$ HAV or HBV acute infection, $2 =$ HBV or HCV carrier) $+ 0.056 \times$ total bilirubin (mg/dL) $- 0.014 \times$ blood choline esterase activity (U/L)
Fulminant hepatitis is likely if prothrombin time <40 % and Z value <0

HAV: hepatitis A virus, HBV: hepatitis B virus, HCV: hepatitis C virus

32.1.2 Other Liver Diseases Treated by Apheresis

Acute fatty liver of pregnancy, Reye's syndrome, acute liver failure caused by impaired hepatic circulation (intrahepatic cholestasis type), and post-surgery acute liver failure can be treated by apheresis. Post-surgery acute liver failure is characterized by relatively lower increases of hepatic enzyme levels, but progressively elevated levels of bilirubin at 7–10 days after surgery. Presurgical liver dysfunction, massive blood loss in surgery, hypotension, infection, and heart failure are other risk factors for acute liver failure.

32.2 Effects of Apheresis on Liver Failure

Yoshiba and colleagues first reported the effect of plasma exchange (PE) plus hemodiafiltration (HDF) on fulminant hepatitis. Among 27 cases, 25 patients showed improvement of unconsciousness and their survival rate was 60 % [2].Of note, this cohort did not include any liver transplantation. Since then, HDF has frequently been used for fulminant hepatitis cases in Japan. Possibly because of a relatively frequent indication of HDF for fulminant hepatitis, the survival rate in the Japanese national survey increased to 40–50 %, while that of the subacute type remains as low as 20–30 % [3]. Sadahiro and colleagues reported that the side effects caused by large amounts of fresh frozen plasma, as described later, were reduced by the addition of HDF [4].

32.3   Plasma Exchange and Hemodiafiltration for Liver Failure

32.3.1   Modality of Apheresis for Liver Failure

PE and PE + hemodialysis (PE + HD) are the most widely used apheresis treatments. These apheresis treatments not only remove bilirubin and molecules that will cause hepatic coma, but also resupply coagulation factors that are reduced by decreased liver synthesis. PE is reportedly performed on more than 90 % of fulminant hepatitis cases in Japan [3]. When the plasma volume for apheresis is above 3.0–3.5 l, tandem-arrayed hemodialysis is conducted to correct metabolic alkalosis and hypocalcemia caused by the large amount of fresh frozen plasma supplementation.

HDF is performed to remove molecules that cause hepatic coma that cannot be sufficiently eliminated by PE. HDF started to be involved for the treatment of fulminant hepatitis in the 1990s and more than 70 % of such cases were treated by HDF in Japan [3]. HDF can be used either intermittently or continuously. Fulminant hepatitis is often complicated with acute kidney injury, and continuous HDF (CHDF) will allow for the control of fluid overload or the removal of humoral mediators including cytokines. A combination of a slow PE, with an exchange of plasma lasting as long as 6–8 h, and high flow CHDF, is also applied in some limited situations.

32.3.2   Indication and Frequency

Apheresis can be reimbursed for fulminant hepatitis, acute liver failure, and post-surgery liver failure under the Japanese insurance system. Only acute liver failure that is as severe as fulminant hepatitis with symptoms of prolonged prothrombin time, coma, and elevated total bilirubin levels will be indicated. Post-surgery liver failure needs at least 2 criteria of total bilirubin levels above 5 mg/dL, hepaplatin test below 40 %, and coma above grade II.

PE is usually performed three to four times per week based on the results of blood tests including prothrombin time and total bilirubin level. The Japanese insurance system limits apheresis treatment sessions for fulminant hepatitis to approximately ten, and that for acute liver failure and post-surgery liver failure to approximately seven.

32.4   Liver Transplantation on Fluminant Hepatitis

Liver transplantation can be performed not only for liver cirrhosis and hepatic cell carcinoma, but for fulminant hepatitis as well since 2004 in Japan. While transplantation has remarkably improved the prognosis of fulminant hepatitis, apheresis as artificial liver support (ALS) also plays an important role as a bridging therapy. It should be noted that a lack of donors is one of the most serious problems for transplantations in Japan. Among the 25 patients with fulminant hepatitis who were referred to the transplant unit of our university hospital (Tokyo University Hospital) in 2008, only 2 patients received liver transplantation. Eight of the patients survived with ALS, while 4 patients who could not be referred for transplantation due to multiple organ failure or deep coma, and 11 patients who could not find any donor candidate for living-related liver transplantation, did not survive.

32.5   Side Effects of Apheresis for Liver Diseases

Side effects of plasma exchange include hypernatremia, metabolic alkalosis, and acute lung edema due to rapid colloid osmotic pressure elevation. Side effects of hemodiafiltration include metabolic acidosis caused by to the use of lactate- or acetic acid-based buffers. The metabolism of lactate and acetate are remarkably reduced in severe liver failure.

Note: Albumin Dialysis
Uremic toxins that accumulate in renal failure are mostly hydrophilic and therefore are effectively removed by hemodialysis. In contrast, only limited toxins in liver failure are hydrophilic and all the other toxins bind to blood albumin. To remove the albumin-bound toxins in liver failure, technicians may use albumin dialysis with the molecular adsorbents recirculating system (MARS®) and fractionated plasma separation and absorption (Prometheus®). MARS employs an albumin solution as the dialysate and can selectively remove albumin-bound toxins [5]. Prometheus removes albumin-bound toxins after separating the plasma and can eliminate hydrophilic toxins by using high-performance dialysis membranes [6]. These apheresis treatments have been widely introduced to clinics in several countries in Asia and Europe, however, they are not available in Japan. This is possibly because applications of PE and HDF for fulminant hepatitis were originally developed in Japan.

References

1. Yoshiba M, Sekiyama K, Inoue K, Yamada M, Kako M, Nagai K, Takatori M, Iwabuchi S, Sumino Y, Tanaka K, Hakozaki Y, Hasegawa K, Shibuya A (2002) Accurate prediction of fulminant hepatic failure in severe acute viral hepatitis: multicenter study. J Gastroenterol 37:916–21
2. Yoshiba M, Sekiyama K, Iwamura Y, Sugata F (1993) Development of reliable artificial liver support (ALS)–plasma exchange in combination with hemodiafiltration using high-performance membranes. Dig Dis Sci 38:469–76
3. Takikawa Y, Suzuki K (2008) Clinical epidemiology of fulminant hepatitis in Japan. Hepatol Res 38:S14–S18
4. Sadahiro T, Hirasawa H, Oda S, Shiga H, Nakanishi K, Kitamura N, Hirano T (2001) Usefulness of plasma exchange plus continuous

hemodiafiltration to reduce adverse effects associated with plasma exchange in patients with acute liver failure. Crit Care Med 29:1386–92

5. Boyle M, Kurtovic J, Bihari D, Riordan S, Steiner C (2004) Equipment review: the molecular adsorbents recirculating system (MARS). Crit Care 8:280–6
6. Falkenhagen D, Strobl W, Vogt G, Schrefl A, Linsberger I, Gerner FJ, Schoenhofen M (1999) Fractionated plasma separation and adsorption system: a novel system for blood purification to remove albumin bound substances. Artif Organs 23:81–6

Chapter 33
Thrombotic Thrombocytopenic Purpura and Thrombotic Microangiopathy

Kenjiro Honda and Kent Doi

Main Points

- Plasma exchange (PE) should be immediately undergone in the probable cases of thrombotic thrombocytopenic purpura (TTP)/thrombotic microangiopathy (TMA) with thrombocytopenia, erythrocyte fragmentation, and hemolytic anemia.
- Replacement of 1–1.5 times the plasma volume with fresh frozen plasma (FFP) during a single procedure of PE is appropriate. PE should be continued until recovery of appropriate laboratory test values and resolution of neurological symptoms, usually after daily PE for 3–5 days.

K. Honda (✉)
Department of Nephrology and Endocrinology, University Hospital,
The University of Tokyo, 7-3-1 Hongo, Bunkyo-ku, Tokyo 113-8655, Japan
e-mail: khonda-tky@umin.ac.jp

K. Doi
Department of Emergency and Critical Care Medicine, University Hospital,
The University of Tokyo, 7-3-1 Hongo, Bunkyo-ku, Tokyo 113-8655, Japan

E. Noiri and N. Hanafusa (eds.), *The Concise Manual*
of Apheresis Therapy, DOI 10.1007/978-4-431-54412-8_33,
© Springer Japan 2014

343

- The effectiveness of PE is controversial, especially in
  O157-induced hemolytic-uremic syndrome (HUS)/
  TMA in children.

33.1   Introduction

Thrombotic thrombocytopenic purpura (TTP) and hemolytic-uremic syndrome (HUS) are acute, fulminant disorders
characterized by hemolytic anemia with erythrocyte fragmentation, thrombocytopenia, and renal impairment.
Although TTP and HUS are often indistinguishable, TTP is
often accompanied by neurologic abnormalities (commonly
with mental status changes) while HUS typically involves
renal dysfunction (see Table 33.1). Thrombotic microangiopathy (TMA) is an inclusive term that describes the morphologic changes of the microvasculature seen in both TTP and
HUS. However, TMA cannot be used synonymously for TTP
and HUS because TMA is also caused by pregnancy and
malignant hypertension. TMA caused by TTP and HUS is
described in this section.

Patients with TTP/TMA had a high mortality rate, exceeding 90 %, before plasma exchange (PE) was introduced. PE
with fresh frozen plasma (FFP) as a replacement solution
improved the mortality rate to <20 %. Recent studies revealed
low activity of ADAMTS-13 (a disintegrin and metalloproteinase with thrombospondin type 1 motifs 13), which is a von
Willebrand factor (vWF) -cleaving protease, in many patients
with TTP/TMA. It was also reported that the activity was
almost normal in patients with HUS/TMA developed from
infection with *Escherichia coli*.

TABLE 33.1 Comparison between TTP and HUS

	TTP	HUS
Age at onset	More common in adult	More common in children
Manifestations	Moschcowitz's pentad Thrombocytopenia, hemolytic anemia, fever, renal dysfunction, and fluctuating neurologic status	Gasser's triad Triad of hemolytic anemia, thrombocytopenia, and acute kidney injury
Characteristics	Neurological symptoms are common in but renal dysfunction is relatively rare	Renal dysfunction is common in but thrombocytopenia is milder
ADAMTS-13	Decreased enzyme activity and presence of its inhibitor	Occasionally decreased enzyme activity but absence of its inhibitor

TTP thrombotic thrombocytopenic purpura, *HUS* hemolytic-uremic syndrome

33.2 Classification of TTP/TMA and HUS/TMA

According to disease development, both TTP/TMA and HUS/TMA are classified into congenital type and acquired type (See Table 33.2). In cases with TTP/TMA, vWF adhesion on platelets has been known to occur.

A multimeric glycoprotein, vWF promotes platelet adhesion and aggregation and is a carrier for Factor VIII in plasma. High molecular weight vWF multimers that are released from vascular endothelial cells promote thrombus formation via platelet aggregation. In a normal state, the high molecular weight vWF multimers are specifically cleaved by a metalloprotease, ADAMTS-13, which prevents abnormal thrombus formation. Reducing ADAMTS-13 activity leads to a significant augmentation of platelet aggregation, which then results in an impairment of microcirculation and the development of TTP/TMA [1]. The pathogenesis associated with the production of

TABLE 33.2 ADAMTS-13 involvement according to cause of TMA

	Cause	Involvement of ADAMTS-13
Congenital TMA	Upshaw–Schulman syndrome	Significantly decreased ADAMTS-13 activity, absence of ADAMTS-13 inhibitor
Acquired TMA	Idiopathic TTP	Decreased ADAMTS-13 activity, most cases with ADAMTS-13 inhibitor
	Drug-induced TTP (ticlopidine/ clopidogrel)	Decreased ADAMTS-13 activity, most cases with ADAMTS-13 inhibitor
	Drug-induced TTP (quinine, mitomycin C, cyclosporine, tacrolimus)	Unknown
	Malignant tumor	Some cases with decreased ADAMTS-13 activity and presence of ADAMTS-13 inhibitor
	Hematopoietic stem cell transplantation	Almost normal ADAMTS-13 activity (some cases with mildly decreased ADAMTS-13 activity)
	Autoimmune disease (SLE, etc.)	Some cases with decreased ADAMTS-13 activity and presence of ADAMTS-13 inhibitor
	Idiopathic HUS	Normal or mildly decreased ADAMTS-13 activity in typical cases
	Enterohemorrhagic *Escherichia coli* (O157) infection	Normal or mildly decreased ADAMTS-13 activity in typical cases

TTP thrombotic thrombocytopenic purpura, *HUS* hemolytic-uremic syndrome, *TMA* thrombotic microangiopathy, *ADAMTS*-13 a disintegrin and metalloproteinase with thrombospondin type 1 motifs 13, *SLE* systemic lupus erythematosus autoantibodies (inhibitors) against ADAMTS-13 is called typical TTP. Typical TTP is classified into primary/idiopathic, and secondary like ticlopidine/clopidogrel-associated TTP [2]. Alternatively, decreased ADAMTS-13 activity and the presence of anti-ADAMTS-13 autoantibodies are not found in the atypical TTP that is associated with hematopoietic stem cell transplantation or malignant tumors. Collagen disease or pregnancy can induce both typical and atypical TTP.

In Upshaw–Schulman syndrome, a congenital TTP, a genetic abnormality causes significantly decreased ADAMTS-13 activity, and FFP transfusion is known as an effective enzyme replacement therapy.

In contrast, both decreased ADAMTS-13 activity and the effectiveness of PE therapy are generally absent in HUS/TMA caused by infection with enterohemorrhagic *E. coli*, O157. Vascular endothelial cell damage due to *E. coli* –produced verotoxin is mainly considered as a cause of typical HUS. When verotoxin binds to globotriaosylceramide (Gb3) located on vascular endothelial cells, large amounts of various inflammatory cytokines are released locally, and then Gb3-rich vascular endothelial cells, especially in the kidney and brain, are damaged. Moreover, activated platelets together with impaired endothelial cells contribute to microthrombus formation and thrombocytopenia.

Excess complement activation due to a genetic abnormality of complement regulatory protein such as H factor, I factor, and membrane cofactor protein has been recently reported to develop recurrent thrombosis in adult HUS without diarrhea. The disease, called familial HUS, comprises 5–10 % of HUS cases.

33.3 Plasma Exchange in TTP/TMA

In a randomized controlled study of PE and FFP transfusion in TTP/TMA cases conducted by Rock et al., remission and survival rates at 6 months were both 78 % in a PE group, while they were 31 % and 50 %, respectively, in a FFP transfusion group [3]. This report revealed the advantage of

PE, although another report showed that the volume of transfused plasma in a PE group was three times as much as in a FFP transfusion group. The superiority of PE may not be explained by the therapeutic efficacy of plasma removal, but rather by the larger amounts of plasma transfused [4]. It has also been shown that the survival rate in ticlopidine-associated TTP/TMA was 50–60 % in PE groups, whereas it was approximately 20 % in non-PE groups [5, 6].

However, the effectiveness of PE is controversial, especially in O157-induced HUS/TMA in children. In these cases, PE should not be frequently performed because of the possibility of volume overload and unknown infection.

33.3.1   ADAMTS-13 in TTP/TMA

PE is only proven to be effective for treatment of TTP/TMA. In typical TTP, its effectiveness is supported by the removal of both ADAMTS-13 inhibitors and high molecular weight vWF multimers, and replacement of both ADAMTS-13 and normal vWF. In contrast, the removal of high molecular weight vWF multimers and replacement of normal vWF may contribute to the treatment of atypical TTP without ADAMTS-13 inhibitors. In the present clinical setting, prompt measurement of ADAMTS-13 activity and its inhibitor titers is difficult, therefore PE is performed soon after the diagnosis of TTP/TMA. Furthermore, PE should be started immediately in those patients with thrombocytopenia, erythrocyte fragmentation, and hemolytic anemia that are unlikely to be caused by other pathologic conditions because emergency treatment is necessary for TTP.

33.3.2   Methods of Plasma Exchange

Replacement of 1–1.5 times the plasma volume with FFP during a single procedure of PE is appropriate. PE is usually recommended to continue until recovery of laboratory test values and resolution of neurologic symptoms, which usually occurs after daily PE for 3–5 days. The measure of treatment effect is normalization of platelet count and lactate dehydrogenase (LDH) levels and the resolution of anemia and neurological symptoms. Several sessions of PE are usually added after the markers of normalization and recovery are seen.

33.3.3 Platelet Transfusion

Platelet transfusion is generally avoided in TMA because it may induce new microthrombus formation and exacerbate nervous system manifestations and kidney damage. Especially in the typical TTP cases with markedly reduced ADAMTS-13 activity, platelet transfusion before PE therapy should be avoided. However, the Oklahoma TTP-HUS registry reported no association between platelet transfusion and worsening of clinical condition. Thus, it may be possible to carefully perform platelet transfusion to prevent bleeding or before invasive treatment [7].

33.4 Differential Diagnosis of TTP/TMA

Thrombotic microvascular damage with thrombocytopenia, hemolytic anemia, and renal dysfunction should be considered in the differential diagnosis of TTP as well as that of HUS (see Table 33.3). In some cases of vasculitis with malignant hypertension and renal impairment, autoantibodies against ADAMTS-13 are present, which makes it difficult to distinguish from idiopathic TTP/TMA. Catastrophic antiphospholipid syndrome shows similar manifestations to TTP, but a prolongation of aPTT and the presence of antiphospholipid autoantibodies help in making the diagnosis. Disseminated intravascular coagulation (DIC) may be part of the differential diagnosis. The pathogenesis of TTP is predominantly the development of platelet thrombosis and platelet consumption, while that of DIC is fibrin thrombus formation followed by activation of the coagulation system. The two diseases can be differentiated by the presence of an activation of the coagulation system.

TABLE 33.3 Differential diagnosis TTP/TMA

Vasculitis
Autoimmune disease (SLE, Rheumatoid arthritis)
Catastrophic antiphospholipid syndrome
Scleroderma renal crisis
Malignant hypertension
DIC (secondary to sepsis, toxemia of pregnancy, etc.)

TTP thrombotic thrombocytopenic purpura, TMA thrombotic microangiopathy, *SLE* systemic lupus erythematosus, *DIC* disseminated intravascular coagulation

Note: Pathogenesis of TTP/TMA

ADAMTS-13 activity has been considered as the main cause of TTP since the enzyme was identified, and high titers of ADAMTS-13 autoantibodies in the acute phase were reported to be a risk factor for recurrence. However, the association between the titers and the responsiveness to PE therapy is controversial. In TTP secondary to drug or malignancy, a decrease in ADAMTS-13 activity and the appearance of its inhibitor are frequently absent even in the acute phase, and PE is not effective as well. However, in those cases with significant decreases of ADAMTS-13 activity and an increase of its inhibitor titer, improvement of the abnormalities in laboratory test values are typically seen with treatment such as corticosteroid administration and PE. The recurrence rate is relatively high in the cases that do not show an improvement of decreased ADAMTS-13 activity and have increases in its inhibitor titer despite recovery from thrombocytopenia and hemolytic anemia after treatment. At present, not all of the pathogenesis is explainable solely by ADAMTS-13 activity. Hence, further investigation is needed.

References

1. Furlan M, Robles R, Galbusera M et al (1998) von Willebrand factor-cleaving protease in thrombotic thrombocytopenic purpura and the hemolytic-uremic syndrome. N Engl J Med 339: 1578–84
2. Scheiflinger F, Knöbl P, Trattner B et al (2003) Nonneutralizing IgM and IgG antibodies to von Willebrand factor-cleaving protease (ADAMTS-13) in a patient with thrombotic thrombocytopenic purpura. Blood 102:3241–3
3. Rock GA, Shumak KH, Buskard NA et al (1991) Comparison of plasma exchange with plasma infusion in the treatment of thrombotic thrombocytopenic purpura. Canadian Apheresis Study Group. N Engl J Med 325:393–7
4. Novitzky N, Jacobs P, Rosenstrauch W (1994) The treatment of thrombotic thrombocytopenic purpura: plasma infusion or exchange? Br J Haematol 87:317–20
5. Bennett CL, Weinberg PD, Rozenberg-Ben-Dror K et al (1998) Thrombotic thrombocytopenic purpura associated with ticlopidine. A review of 60 cases. Ann Intern Med 128:541–4
6. Bennett CL, Davidson CJ, Raisch DW et al (1999) Thrombotic thrombocytopenic purpura associated with ticlopidine in the setting of coronary artery stents and stroke prevention. Arch Intern Med 159:2524–8
7. Swisher KK, Terrell DR, Vesely SK et al (2009) Clinical outcomes after platelet transfusions in patients with thrombotic thrombocytopenic purpura. Transfusion 49:873–87

Chapter 34
Inflammatory Bowel Diseases

Tsuyoshi Inoue

Main Points
- Apheresis to remove leukocytes from peripheral blood is a treatment option for inflammatory bowel diseases.
- Apheresis to remove leukocytes has been proposed as a feasible, safe, and effective therapy.

34.1 Introduction

Ulcerative colitis (UC) and Crohn's disease (CD) are the representative disorders of inflammatory bowel diseases (IBD).UC normally involves a continuous area from the rectum to the colon while CD may affect any part of the gastrointestinal tract from the mouth to the anus.Mild forms of

T. Inoue (✉)

Division of Nephrology and Endocrinology, School of Medicine,
The University of Tokyo, 7-3-1 Hongo, Bunkyo-ku, Tokyo 113-8655, Japan
e-mail: tsinoue-tky@umin.ac.jp

E. Noiri and N. Hanafusa (eds.), *The Concise Manual*
of Apheresis Therapy, DOI 10.1007/978-4-431-54412-8_34,
© Springer Japan 2014

IBD are usually successfully treated with aminosalicylates (Pentasa®) for maintenance of remission and with corticosteroids for flares. Management of moderate and severe forms of IBD is far from being fully satisfactory, especially for the many cases of steroid dependency, steroid resistance, and steroid intolerance. A large number of different therapeutic approaches have been tried in the last decade. Among them, apheresis for removal of leukocytes from peripheral blood by using extracorporeal circulation has been proposed as a feasible, safe, and effective therapy for IBD.

34.2   Ulcerative Colitis

UC is associated with chronic relapsing inflammation of the mucosal layer of the colon. UC normally involves a continuous area from the rectum to the colon, with the rectum almost universally being involved.

34.2.1   Therapeutic Targets (Objects and Medical Conditions)

34.2.1.1   Targeted Objects

The targets of apheresis in IBD are leukocytes, including granulocytes, monocytes, and lymphocytes.

34.2.1.2   Etiology

Clinical conditions differ between UC and CD, the representative diseases of IBD. Although the cause of IBD is unknown, a crucial pathogenic role is attributed to leukocytes. Activated granulocytes and monocytes represent the major source of pro-inflammatory cytokines in the intestinal mucosa and play a pivotal role in inducing and maintaining intestinal inflammation. Apheresis to remove activated leukocytes from peripheral blood by using extracorporeal circulation can ameliorate the clinical conditions of IBD. Apheresis is also reported to increase levels of anti-inflammation cytokines [1]. Taking these facts into account, we can presume that this treatment effect is acting through multiple mechanisms.

34.2.2   Effect of the Treatment

GCAP (granulocytapheresis) was applied to patients with UC who were refractory to conventional or steroid therapy and many clinical studies have shown that this treatment is effective among 40–100 % of patients [2]. In regards to leukocytapheresis (LCAP),66.6–100 % of the patients with active UC achieved clinical remission with LCAP [2], including an 80 % achievement rate shown in a double-blind, multicenter prospective study [3]. Recently, intensive apheresis (twice a week) in patients with active UC was reported to be more efficacious than weekly treatment [4]. Furthermore, even among pediatric UC patients, apheresis was shown to be effective for reducing the number of leukocytes [2].

34.3   Crohn's Disease

CD may affect any part of the gastrointestinal tract from the mouth to the anus. In most cases, the affected site is limited to the ileum, ileum and cecum, or ileum and whole colon, and inflammation of the stomach or upper gastrointestinal tract occurs in approximately 30 % of the patients.

34.3.1   Therapeutic Targets (Objects and Medical Conditions)

34.3.1.1   Targeted Objects

The targets of apheresis in CD are leukocytes including granulocytes, monocytes, and lymphocytes.

34.3.1.2   Etiology

See the section on UC.

34.3.2   Effect of the Treatment

Five of the seven patients with active CD who were refractory to conventional treatments were reported to achieve remission by GCAP [5], and 52–83 % of patients in other studies with a similar background responded to the treatment [2]. The reports concerning LCAP are limited, but there is a report that 9 of 18 patients (50 %) achieved clinical remission with the LCAP procedure [6].

34.4   Therapeutic Protocol

34.4.1   The Selection of the Treatment

To date, two methods (LCAP or GCAP) are available for selective leukocytapheresis in patients with IBD. The biggest difference between them is the type of cells that can be removed. Both methods can remove the granulocytes and monocytes, but only LCAP can remove lymphocytes induced by chronic inflammation. The conditions for removing pro-inflammatory cytokines differ in the two methods, so it is necessary to choose the method by considering the patient's medical condition and evidence, but there is currently no standard for the selection of the method. Centrifugal leukocytapheresis is also available and only needs one venous access. However, this requires a specialized machine for the treatment, so this method has not become popular.

34.4.2   Extracorporeal Circulation

Neither therapy requires high blood flow, so the treatment only needs two venous access points with 18-gauge needles, e.g., one access site at the antecubital (or femoral) vein on one arm for blood supply into the equipment and one access on the other arm for returning the blood to the patient.

34.4.3   Anticoagulants

Nafamostat mesylate or heparin are used to prevent coagulation of blood during the extracorporeal circulation. Nafamostat mesylate is the first choice because of the risk for bleeding of the gastrointestinal tract. However, there is a report that the use of heparin was associated with a significantly lower frequency of adverse events such as coagulation of blood as compared to the rate seen with nafamostat mesylate [7].

34.4.4   Treatment Schedule

The standard schedule is once weekly for 5 consecutive weeks (one course). In patients who do not response well to one course of treatment, another course (a total of ten sessions) can be provided. In addition, different protocols with two sessions per week or other schedules have also been tested.

34.5   Modality

A comparison of LCAP and GCAP for selective leukocytapheresis in patients with IBD in shown in Table 34.1.

Centrifugal leukocytapheresis is also available in addition to the methods shown in the table.

34.6   Safety Precaution

34.6.1   Exacerbation of Infection

Any existing infection can become worse because of the decreased number of white blood cells. GCAP treatment is

TABLE 34.1 Leukocytapheresis and granulocytapheresis for inflammatory bowel diseases

LCAP(leukocytapheresis)

• Equipment	Cellsorba® (Asahi Medical, Tokyo, Japan)
• Duration per session	Blood flow rate 30–50 mL/min for 60 min

> The Cellsorba leukocyte removal filter is made of polyester fibers that are able to remove a large amount of white blood cells, about 90–100 % of granulocytes and monocytes, 30–60 % of lymphocytes. In addition, a certain amount of platelets (30 % in the first 30 min of the session) from peripheral blood are also removed

GCAP(granulocytapheresis)

• Equipment	Adacolumn® (Japan Immunoresearch Laboratories Co., Ltd)
• Duration per session	Blood flow rate 30 mL/min for 60 min

> The apheresis column filled with 2–3 mm diameter cellulose acetate beads that act as selective adsorptive carriers for granulocytes and monocytes, but not for lymphocytes and platelets (The carriers adsorb about 60 % of the granulocytes and monocytes/macrophages and only 2 % of lymphocytes)

contraindicated for patients whose granulocyte count is <2,000/mm^3. For patients with <3,000/mm^3 white blood cells, LCAP treatment can be provided with care.

34.6.2 Coagulation of Blood During Extracorporeal Circulation

Compared to that seen in other methods of apheresis, the blood flow in LCAP and GCAP is slow, and the circuit should be monitored for signs of coagulation. To prevent coagulation of the blood in LCAP, a syringe of an anticoagulant agent is connected to the blood circuit line just before the point where the blood enters the column. Even with anticoagulant therapy, the frequency of coagulation of the blood in LCAP is higher than seen in GCAP.

34.6.3   Hypotension

Extracorporeal circulation of the blood can cause hypotension. Hypotension is sometimes associated with dehydration due to continuous diarrhea, and in that case, 100–200 mL normal saline should be administrated via the blood circuit line. In patients with abnormalities of the gastrointestinal tract who are undergoing apheresis, hypotension resulting from dehydration can cause an exacerbation of digestive tract symptoms, especially those concerning bowel movements. It is important to carefully monitor such patients to prevent the development of hypotension. Vagal reflex and a drug allergy to nafamostat mesylate may also cause hypotension (See also Chap. 17: hypotension section).

34.6.4   Other Side Effects

An allergic reaction to nafamostat mesylate can induce anaphylactic shock.

Note: The Future of the Apheresis for Removal of Leukocytes
GCAP and LCAP for treatment of IBD, therapeutic methods that originated in Japan, are now widely performed in many countries and regions. However, evidence to support these methods of treatment are limited, and the exact indications have not been established. Future elucidation of the pathologic mechanism of IBD and the results of larger randomized controlled trials are awaited.

References

1. Yagi Y et al (2007) Ther Apher Dial 11:331–336
2. Danese S et al (2008) Digestion 77:96–107
3. Sawada K et al (2005) Am J Gastroenterol 100:1362–1369
4. Sakuraba A et al (2009) Am J Gastroenterol 104:2990–2995
5. Matsui T et al (2003) Am J Gastroenterol 98:511–512
6. Kosaka T et al (1999) Intern Med 38:102–111
7. Ashizuka S et al (2006) Ther Apher Dial 10:54–58

Chapter 35
Hepatitis C Virus Infection

Shi Lu and Eisei Noiri

Main Points
- The indications for apheresis are hepatitis C virus (HCV) serotype 1 cases with HCV-RNA more than 100 kIU/mL and interferon-α (IFN) resistive.
- Plasma fractionator (2nd filter) of double filtration plasmapheresis (DFPP) is equivalent to Cascadeflo™ EC-50 W with a size pore of 30 nm.
- Immediately after DFPP, HCV starts showing a rebound phenomenon. The timing of IFN administration has to be as soon as possible.
- When patients have a history of splenectomy, catheter infection tends to cause severe septicemia.

S. Lu • E. Noiri (✉)
Department of Hemodialysis & Apheresis, University Hospital,
The University of Tokyo, 7-3-1 Hongo, Bunkyo-ku, Tokyo 113-8655, Japan
e-mail: noiri-tky@umin.ac.jp

E. Noiri and N. Hanafusa (eds.), *The Concise Manual
of Apheresis Therapy*, DOI 10.1007/978-4-431-54412-8_35,
© Springer Japan 2014

35.1   Introduction

It has been reported that a reduction of the copy numbers of hepatitis C virus (HCV)-RNA is often seen after hemodialysis therapy [1]. However, the viral load of HCV from the liver is enormous; its generation rate is 10^{12} virions per day and its half life is 2.7 h. Because of this high generation rate, it has been considered unlikely that the blood cleansing effect of double filtration plasmapheresis (DFPP) would be effective enough to keep the HCV level low or even to attain a viral free condition, namely sustained virological response (SVR). A recent report from Japan is overturning these fixed concepts with an intensive prescription of both DFPP and interferon-α (IFN) toward HCV serotype 1 that are resistive to IFN due to higher viral level [2]. Figure 35.1 shows a

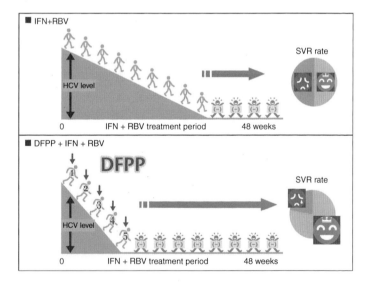

FIGURE 35.1 Concept of virus removal and eradication by double filtration plasmapheresis (VRAD). VRAD includes double filtration plasmapheresis (DFPP) to the regular hepatitis C virus therapy to facilitate reaching and early sustained virological response (SVR). IFN denotes as interferon-α and RBV as ribavirin

schematic interpretation where the combination of DFPP, pegylated-interferon-α (PEG-IFN), and ribavirin (RBV) can decrease the HCV level rapidly compared with regular PEG-IFN and RBV therapy, thus enabling the patient to reach a SVR condition and to achieve complete remission. Figure 35.2 demonstrates the practical efficacy of combined therapy (DFPP + PEG-IFN + RBV), successfully boosting SVR, compared with the regular therapy (PEG-IFN + RBV) [3].

35.2   Virus Removal and Eradication by Double Filtration Plasmapheresis (VRAD)

The DFPP procedure prescribed to eradicate HCV is now called VRAD (virus removal and eradication by DFPP) in Japan [2]. In VRAD, plasma separation is achieved by a plasma separator (1st filter; Plasmaflo™ OP-08 W or equivalent), and 2nd filter (Cascadeflo™ EC-50 W or equivalent) with a size pore of 30 nm preclude the reentrance of viral particles with a diameter of 55–60 nm in theoretical value Fig. 35.3.

The efficacy after VRAD for the reduction of viral load is under the detection limit in almost all cases when plasma was monitored immediately after the 2nd filter at the time points of the half and final therapeutic periods. When the efficacy is monitored in the patients' blood level, HCV viral load reduced from $2,393 \pm 2,139$ kIU/mL in the beginning to $1,494 \pm 969$ kIU/mL at the end of VRAD [3]. Based on the total processed plasma volume $3,161 \pm 421$ mL (mean ± SD), calculated HCV-RNA removal during a single round of DFPP is $3.08 \pm 5.81 \times 10^9$ IU and the removal rate is $26.1\% \pm 36.4\%$. In addition, it is known that a rebound phenomenon is seen a couple of hours after treatment. Immediate IFN treatment after DFPP is ideal to achieve the maximum efficacy of anti-HCV treatment, reduce the chance of reinfection to healthy hepatic cells, minimize the rebound, and to further increase efficacy in subsequent rounds of VRAD. In

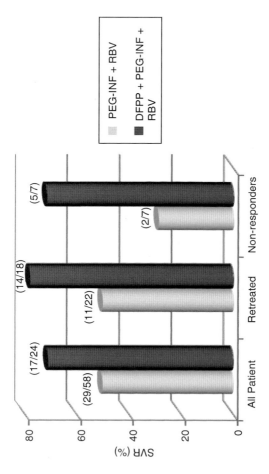

FIGURE 35.2 Sustained virological response (SVR) rate between double filtration plasmapheresis (DFPP) and non-DFPP. Patients consist of an hepatitis C virus (HCV) cohort of non-treated, re-treated, or non-responders to interferon-α (IFN). This figure is from Fujiwara (2008) with modification

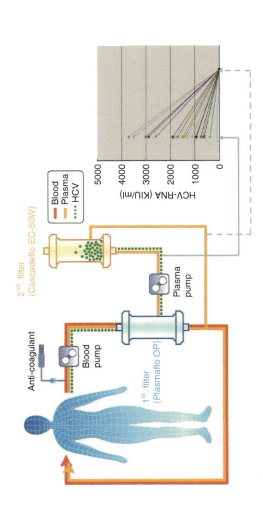

FIGURE 35-3 Scheme of double filtration plasmapheresis in virus removal and eradication by double filtration plasmapheresis (VRAD) efficacy. This figure is from Fujiwara (2008) with modification

patients with chronic hepatitis C infection, there are two fractions of HCV particles in the blood according to its buoyant density, which relates to viral titer or disease states. One is a high-density fraction in which HCV particles form an immunocomplex with immunoglobulin G (IgG), the other is a low-density fraction where HCV particles bind to low-density lipoprotein (LDL). Removal of circulating HCV by DFPP treatment mostly decreases the amount of the high-density fraction of HCV particles, which may be associated with the IFN response [4, 5]. Thus, DFPP plus IFN combination can produce a great reduction of viral load during the early stage of treatment and achieve a high SVR.

However, doctors have to pay attention to the level of fibrinogen. The reduction of fibrinogen is often seen during rounds of DFPP (approximately reduction rate is 38 %), but the occurrence is more common in patients with chronic liver disease. When the fibrinogen level is below 100 mg/dL before DFPP, a delay of DFPP treatment is necessary for that day, but continuation can be considered after a reevaluation of the fibrinogen level. Hypotension and nausea are temporary side effects and are seen at the same frequency as in other DFPP procedures. A double lumen catheter will be placed for blood access for VRAD, usually performed five times during the hospital admission period in Japan (refer to Fig. 35.4). It should be noted that catheter infection tends to cause severe septicemia when patients have a history of splenectomy.

35.3   Typical Protocol

Figure 35.4 shows a typical VRAD protocol. Serum fibrinogen level is a crucial limiting factor for the scheduling of DFPP; a maximum five procedures is recommended. DFPP is usually performed on days 1, 2, 4, 8, and 9, prescribing a plasma processing dose of 50 mL/kg. PEG-IFN is on day 1 and 8 immediately after DFPP (usually within 1 h).

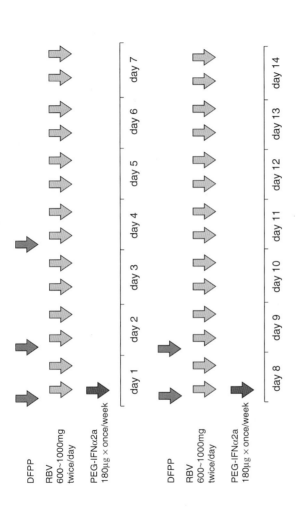

FIGURE 35.4 Protocol of virus removal and eradication by double filtration plasmapheresis (VRAD). After 2 weeks, a regular protocol of hepatitis C virus (HCV) therapy (PEG-IFN + RBV) continues until 48 weeks. IFN denotes as interferon-α, RBV is ribavirin, PEG is pegylated

After 2 weeks, regular protocol of HCV therapy (PEG-IFN + RBV) continues until 48 weeks.

DFPP

RBV
600~1000mg
twice/day

PEG-IFNα2a
180μg × once/week

day 1   day 2   day 3   day 4   day 5   day 6   day 7

DFPP

RBV
600~1000mg
twice/day

PEG-IFNα2a
180μg × once/week

day 8   day 9   day 10   day 11   day 12   day 13   day 14

References

1. Noiri E, Nakao A, Oya A, Fujita T, Kimura S (2001) Hepatitis C virus in blood and dialysate in hemodialysis. Am J Kidney Dis 37:38–42
2. Yamashita T, Arai K, Sakai A, Mizukoshi E, Sakai Y, Kagaya T, Nakamoto Y, Honda M, Wada T, Yokoyama H, Kaneko S (2006) Virological effects and safety of combined double filtration plasmapheresis (DFPP) and interferon therapy in patients with chronic hepatitis C: a preliminary study. Hepatol Res 36:167–175
3. Fujiwara K, Kaneko S, Kakumu S, Sata M, Hige S, Tomita E, Mochida S (2007) Virus Reduction Therapy Study Group: Double filtration plasmapheresis and interferon combination therapy for chronic hepatitis C patients with genotype 1 and high viral load. Hepatol Res 37:701–710
4. Hijikata M, Shimizu YK, Kato H, Iwamoto A, Shih JW, Alter HJ, Purcell RH, Yoshikura H (1993) Equilibrium centrifugation studies of hepatitis C virus: evidence for circulating immune complexes. J Virol 67:1953–1958
5. Omata M, Yokosuka O, Takano S, Kato N, Hosoda K, Imazeki F, Toda M, Ito Y, Ohto M (1991) Resolution of acute hepatitis C after therapy with natural beta interferon. Lancet 338:914–915

Chapter 36
Drug Intoxication

Motonobu Nakamura

> **Main Points**
> - The characteristics of both the offending drugs and the extracorporeal circulation circuit must be understood
> - A brief initial screening examination should be performed on all patients to identify immediate measures required to stabilize and prevent deterioration of their medical condition.

36.1 Introduction

Apheresis therapy may be effective in accidental and intentional poisoning or drug overdose. Especially in Japan, extracorporeal circulation such as plasma exchange (PEx) or hemadsorption can be used for treatment of drug overdose

M. Nakamura (✉)
Department of Nephrology and Endocrinology, Graduate School of Medicine, The University of Tokyo, 7-3-1 Hongo, Bunkyo-ku, Tokyo 113-8655, Japan
e-mail: nakamura-stm@umin.ac.jp

E. Noiri and N. Hanafusa (eds.), *The Concise Manual of Apheresis Therapy,* DOI 10.1007/978-4-431-54412-8_36, © Springer Japan 2014

and poisoning. It is important to evaluate apheresis methods by considering the following three factors:

1. Whether the drug can be removed by extracorporeal circulation.
2. Whether apheresis is an effective or ineffective therapy after considering the risks of extracorporeal circulation.
3. What treatment method will be best for removing the target toxic substance.

36.2   The Target Substances and Pathology

36.2.1   Indication

The indications for extracorporeal circulation are shown in Table 36.1 [1].

36.2.2   The Target Substances

The target substances of extracorporeal circulation are shown in Table 36.2 [2, 3].

TABLE 36.1 Indications for blood purification in drug toxicosis

1. If the general state becomes progressively worse, in spite of having undergone standard treatment.
2. If there is brainstem dysfunction (i.e. respiratory depression, hypotension, hypothermia etc.)
3. If deep coma with pneumonia or sepsis is present
4. If severe organ injury is present that affects the metabolism of the causative agent
5. If the metabolic products of the causative agents have toxicity
6. If the causative agents may cause delayed organ injury

Modified Japanese Society for Clinical Toxicology Guidelines (http://journalsonline.tandf.co.uk/media/f83gxpxyvj02my13xxb0/contributions/t/g/c/q/tgcq8hk3u9xn0e6r.pdf)

TABLE 36.2 The substances that can be removed by various apheresis methods

	Substances	MW	Vd (L/kg)	Protein-binding rate (%)	Clearance (ml/min) Endogenous	HD	HA	Removal rate for 4 hs Endogenous	HD	HA
The substances which can be removed by HD	Alcohol Isopropanol	46								
	Ethanol	46	0.6	0.0	170–320	120–160	(−)	76	87	
	Ethylene glycol	62	0.8	0.0	64	100–200	(−)			
	Methanol	32	0.6	0.0	44	98–176	(−)	22	56	
	Bromide Potassium bromide									
	Distigmine bromide	576								
	Neostigmine bromide	303		15.0						
	Antipsychotics Lithium	7	0.8	0.00	20	150	(−)	8	5	
	Aniline	93								
	Oxalic acid	90								

(continued)

TABLE 36.2 (continued)

Substances		MW	Vd (L/kg)	Protein-binding rate (%)	Clearance(ml/min)			Removal rate for 4 hs		
					Endogenous	HD	HA	Endogenous	HD	HA
Sedative agents	Bromovalerylurea	223	0.7		5	100				
	Chloral hydrate	165	6	35–41	600	120	157–238	29	34	37
NSAIDs	Acetaminophen	151	1	10–21	400	120	125	75	83	83
	Aspirin	180	0.2	73–94	45	20	90	52	65	89
Anti-arrhythmic agents	Atenolol	266	1.2	<5	176	29–39		40	45	
	Sotalol hydrochloride	309	1.2–2.4	~9						
	Procainamide hydrochloride	272	2.9	~15	684				30	
	Disopyramide	339	0.8	5–65	93	123		32	40	
Antibiotics agents	Aminoglycoside									
Pesticide	Boracic acid	62								
	Glufosinate	198			200	40	(−)			

The substances which can be removed by HA		MW	Vd							
Bronchodilating agents	Theophylline	180	0.5	60	46	70	100–125	30	59	74
Sedative agents	Phenobarbital	232	0.8	25–60	9	80	80–290	14	14	61
	Secobarbital Sodium	260								
Antiepileptic agents	Carbamazepine	236	1	70–80	59		80–129	17	17	36
	Phenytoin	252	0.6	87–93	25		76–189	14	14	61
Anti-arrhythmic agents	Lidocaine hydrochloride	234	1.2	66	606	(−)	75–90	82	82	86
Cardiac glycoside	Digitoxin	765	0.5	90	3	(−)	19	2	2	14
Anti-metabolic agents	Methotrexate	454								
Agrichemical agents	Paraquat	186	2.8	50	28	10	57–156			
Mushroom toxin	Amanita toxin									

The blank means no-data

MW molecular weight, *HA* hemadsorption, *HD* hemodialysis, *Vd* volume of distribution

36.2.3 Minimum Requirements

The characteristics of both the offending drugs and the extracorporeal circulation circuit must be understood In particular, it is important to know the molecular weight, protein binding rate, volume of distribution (Vd) and organization shift, half life and endogenous clearance of the offending drugs.

A brief initial screening examination should be performed on all patients to identify immediate measures required to stabilize and prevent deterioration of their medical condition including obtaining vital statistics and measuring electrolyte balance.

1. Molecular weight
   Hemodialysis may be performed if the molecular weight of the substance to be removed is less than 500–2,000 Da. If the molecular weight is 500–40,000 Da, hemofiltration or hemodiafiltration (HDF) may be performed. Hemadsorption can be used to remove substances with molecular weights of 100–10,000 Da.
2. Protein binding rate
   PEx or hemadsorption, but not hemodialysis, is used to remove drugs with high protein binding rates. However, caution is required because PEx or hemadsorption therapies require large amount of blood products, and may cause thrombopenia.
3. Volume of distribution and organization shift
   The Vd equals the total amount of drug in the body divided by the plasma concentration before treatment. In general, if the target drugs are lipid soluble the drug will distribute beyond the plasma and into the tissues and the Vd will be large. Therefore, these substances will have a low concentration in plasma, and may be difficult to remove by extracorporeal circulation.
4. Half-life and endogenous clearance
   Substances with a short half-life will have a high endogenous clearance and blood purification may not be effective for their removal. Moreover, for substances with a short

half-life, it is important to begin apheresis as soon as possible after toxic drug intake. Blood purification methods may be ineffective when a long time has passed since intake of the toxic drug.

36.3   The Choice and Effect of Blood Purification

36.3.1   Hemodialysis, Hemofiltration, Continuous Hemodiafiltration

There is no clear evidence supporting the use of hemodialysis, hemofiltration, or continuous hemodiafiltration (CHDF) for removal of toxic substances. Furthermore, the clearance per unit time is low in CHDF. Therefore, CHDF may be ineffective in rapid removal of toxic substances.

Although there is no clear evidence the use of hemodialysis or hemofiltration, hemodialysis or hemofiltration may be useful in removing some toxins as follow described.

- Low molecular weight
- Small Vd
- Low degree of protein-binding
- High water solubility and low lipid solubility
- Low endogeneous clearance

In the cases of acute kidney injury with drug toxicosis and abnormalities of volume balance or metabolic acidosis, blood purification therapy is needed. If the patient is hemodynamically unstable, CHDF may be the best treatment.

36.3.2   Hemadsorption

Hemadsorption cannot used for a long duration. Therefore drugs with a large Vd or substances with prolonged action may show increased blood concentrations after blood purification therapy has ended.

36.3.3   PEx

In theory, PEx, which is largely unaffected by molecular weight or protein binding rate, may have the largest range of removal of toxic substances. However, PEx has some issues, for example, it requires supplementation with blood products, is expensive, and has a long preparation time. Furthermore PEx has some complications as hypocalcemia. Parestheasis, muscle cramps, nausea, hypotension, and allergic symptoms.

36.4   Indication of Blood Purification in Main Drug Toxicosis

The characteristics of the main drugs or substances are shown in Table 36.2. However, there is little evidence concerning the effect of blood purification on the prognosis of drug toxicosis.

36.4.1   Medicinal Products

(a) Central nervous system drugs
    Most central nervous system drugs have a large Vd and a high protein binding rate. However, because lithium has a low molecular weight and low protein binding rate, hemodialysis may be effective for lithium toxicosis.
(b) Antipyretic and analgetic drugs
    Acetaminophen may cause organ damage (mainly in the liver) with an intake of more than 250 mg/kg, but acetaminophen has a rapid endogenous clearance. Therefore, blood purification may be not effective. However, in the cases of fulminant hepatitis or hepatic failure, PEx and/or hemodiafiltration may be effective.

    There is a report that salicylic acid toxicosis may cause acute kidney injury. Hemodialysis is effective in acute kidney injury, but because salicylic acid has a relatively high protein binding rate, it may not be able to removed by hemodialysis.

(c) Circulatory agents
Digoxin has a high protein binding rate and a large Vd. Therefore, hemodialysis or hemadsorption may be ineffective in digoxin toxicosis. Other circulatory agents, including antihypertensive agents, also have high protein binding rates and large Vds, and the removal efficiency of hemofiltration or hemadsorption may not exceed that of endogenous clearance.

(d) Respiratory agents
In theophylline toxicosis, hemadsorption may be used when the drug concentration exceeds 80 mg per milliliter. However, hemadsorption may be beneficial if the patients have symptoms such as arrhythmia and seizure, even though the concentration is less than 80 mg per milliliter.

(e) Antibiotic agents
Most antibiotics can be removed by hemadsorption. Oral aminoglycoside antibiotics, such as vancomycin, have a lower tendency to cause toxicosis because these agents are poorly absorbed by intestinal tract. However, hemodialysis or hemadsorption can be provided for patients receiving antibiotics administered by the intravenous route.

(f) Metabolic agents
Lactic acidosis is a well-known side effect of toxicosis by biguanide medicines, which are oral antihyperglycemic agents. In patients with lactic acidosis, hemodialysis may be effective.

36.4.2 Chemical Agents

Ethylene glycol, methanol, ethanol, and similar chemical agents can cause toxicosis. These agents may be able to be removed by hemodialysis because these substances have a low molecular weight.

36.4.2.1   Methanol Toxicosis

Diagnostic criteria for methanol toxicosis are serum methanol levels >20 mg/dL ,or plasma osmolal gap >10 mOsm/kg H_2O, or methanol toxicosis strongly suspected from the clinical history (pH < 7.3, HCO_3 < 20 mEq/L). If the patients satisfy two of these criteria, oral ethanol administration (absolute ethanol is diluted with distilled water to 20 %; initial dose is 600 mg/kg and maintenance dose is 66 mg/kg per hour) should be started. In addition, 1 mg/kg of folic acid is administrated to the patient every 4 h. If the patients do not respond to these treatments, or show evidence of end organ damage (i.e. central nervous system damage, renal insufficiency, etc), hemodialysis is the best method to rapidly remove the methanol [4].

36.4.2.2   Ethylene Glycol and Ethanol Toxicosis

If the patients present with a plasma ethanol concentration >20 mg/dL or an osmolal gap >10 mOsm/kg H_2O, they may be given antagonist agents. Ethylene glycol toxicosis may be diagnosed if the patients satisfy two or more of the following signs: a strongly suggestive clinical history; pH < 7.3; HCO_3 level <20 mEq/L; osmolal gap >10 mOsm/kg H_2O; or the presence of oxalic acid crystals in the urine. In Japan, ethanol is the only antagonist agent. If the patients do not respond to this treatment and acidosis is present (pH <7.25–7.3), or they present with acute kidney injury, hemodialysis is the best method to rapidly remove the ethanol (http://journalsonline. tandf.co.uk/media/f83gxpxyvj02my13xxb0/contributions/t/ g/c/q/tgcq8hk3u9xn0e6r.pdf).

36.4.2.3   Agrichemical Agents

There is no clear evidence for the effectiveness of blood purification treatment for poisoning with agrichemical agents. Furthermore, in paraquat toxicosis, paraquat presents a "hit-and-run" type of organ injury whereby the concentration of the drug in the target organ can cause a delayed toxicity. There are no clear data about removing toxic substances with this characteristic.

36.4.2.4   Natural Toxin

Most of the toxicity of mushrooms comes from the amanita toxin. Amanita toxin is removed by hemadsorption. However, it remains unknown whether hemadsorption is effective in the early phase. Symptomatic therapy is provided in the case of the aconite toxin, snake toxin, and tetrodotoxin toxin.

> **Note: MARS (Molecular Adsorbent Recirculating System, MARS®) [5]**
> MARS is a recently reported new blood purification method. In this system albumin (Alb)-binding substances are separated from the blood and then the water-soluble substances are removed by the bicarbonate dialysis fluid. Finally, Alb-binding substances are adsorbed by the activated carbon and ion-exchange resin. Reusing this purified Alb-floating fluid has proved to be efficacious. Although this system has a high cost and a relatively complicated circuit, it is able to remove even Alb-binding substances. Therefore, this method may become a new blood purification system in drug toxicosis.

References

1. Japanese Society for clinical toxicology. @http://jsct.umin.jp/page041.html
2. Owen HG, Brecher ME (1994) Transfusion 34(10):891–894
3. Pond SM (1984) Emerg Med Clin North Am 2:29–45
4. Barceloux DG, Bond GR et al (2002) J Toxicol Clin Toxicol 40: 415–446
5. de Pont AC (2007) Curr Opin Crit Care 13:668–673

Chapter 37
Living Related Kidney Transplantation

Hiroo Kawarazaki

Main Points
- Therapeutic apheresis is one of the key perioperative strategies for reduction of antibodies directed against donor antigens such as anti-ABO blood type antibody or anti-donor specific human leukocyte antigen (HLA) antibody. Simultaneous therapeutic apheresis can improve kidney survival in antibody mediated rejection.

37.1 Introduction

Japan has very few deceased kidney donors and therefore, as a means to increase the demands of kidney transplantation, ABO-incompatible transplantation (see Notes) was started since 1989. Now, ABO-incompatible kidney transplantation

H. Kawarazaki (✉)
Department of Internal Medicine, Division of Nephrology
and Hypertension, Kawasaki 2-16-1, Sugao, Miyamae-ku 216-8511, Japan
e-mail: hirookawarazaki@yahoo.co.jp

E. Noiri and N. Hanafusa (eds.), *The Concise Manual of Apheresis Therapy,* DOI 10.1007/978-4-431-54412-8_37,
© Springer Japan 2014

382   H. Kawarazaki

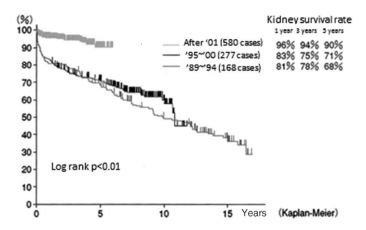

FIGURE 37.1 Comparison of kidney survival between eras

accounts for about 15 % of all living related kidney transplantation in Japan, which has become a leading country in the practice of ABO-incompatible kidney transplantation. Due to the innovation of therapeutic immunosuppression, kidney survival after ABO-incompatible kidney transplantation has favorable results similar to that for ABO-compatible kidney transplantation [1] (Fig. 37.1). In the ABO-incompatible recipient, anti-A or -B antibodies directed against the ABO antigen expressed in the intima of the donor renal artery are the cause of humoral rejection. Likewise, pre-formed or newly-formed donor specific HLA antibodies are the cause of humoral rejection in HLA-antibody related rejection. Elimination of such antibodies, called desensitization, is the purpose of therapeutic apheresis in kidney transplantation and has an essential role together with immunosuppressive therapy. Because ABO-incompatible kidney transplantation needs patient desensitization before transplantation, ABO-incompatible transplantation is not indicated for deceased donor kidney transplantation.

37.2   Apheresis Before Transplantation

37.2.1   ABO-Incompatible Transplantation

37.2.1.1   Target of Elimination and Pathophysiology

Target: Anti-A or -B IgG, IgM antibody.
Pathophysiology: Anti-A or -B antibodies directed against donor vascular endothelium.

37.2.1.2   Therapeutic Effect

Removing as many anti-A or -B antibodies as possible is favored. Many institutions aim to reduce antibody titer level below 16–32 after apheresis.

37.2.1.3   Treatment

Insurance restrictions: four timest before and two times after transplantation
Modality: Plasma exchange (PE) and double filter plasmapheresis (DFPP) are indicated. Plasma adsorption is also possible but at the moment is not covered by insurance. The characteristics of PE and DFPP are shown in Table 37.1 [2], and the therapeutic plasma exchange volume is usually 1.2–1.5 times the plasma volume.

TABLE 37.1   Characteristics of therapeutic apheresis

	Plasma exchange	Double filter plasmapheresis
Replacement fluid	Fresh frozen plasma	Albumin and saline
Coagulation factors	No change	Reduction
Allergic reaction	Mild risk	Low risk
Risk of infection	Mild risk	Low risk
Others	Citrate intoxication Hypocalcemia	Hypoglobulinemia

Actual frequency: Depending on the titer of the antibodies of the target, two to three times before transplantation is common. In our institution, DFPP is done between dialysis sessions. On the day before transplantation either PE, or DFPP with the addition of ten units of fresh frozen plasma to restore coagulation factors, is done followed by hemodialysis.

Therapeutic target: In most institutions, an anti-A or -B titer below 16–32 times is preferred. Due to innovations in immunosuppression, recipients with high titers can be desensitized and safely undergo transplantation treatment [3]. However, recipients showing high titer rebound after apheresis are at risk of acute antibody mediated rejection. In such patients, sufficient immunosuppression and frequent apheresis (as many as ten times) before transplantation may be indicated.

37.2.1.4   Points to Note

When DFPP is chosen, discarded plasma must be replaced by albumin and normal saline. When PE is chosen, plasma must be replaced by blood type AB plasma that contains no anti-A or -B antibodies.

37.2.2   Anti-Donor Specific HLA Antibody Positive Transplantation

37.2.2.1   Target of Elimination and Pathophysiology

Target: Mainly anti-donor specific HLA IgG antibodies.
Pathophysiology: Anti-donor specific HLA antibodies directed against donor kidney.

37.2.2.2   Therapeutic Effect

Recipients of positive direct T cell complement dependent cytotoxic (CDC) crossmatch tests are contraindicated for transplantation. However, a negative direct T cell CDC but a positive crossmatch test with flow cytometry, a highly sensitive marker, may enable transplantation (see Notes). The criteria for successful transplantation in such circumstances are not standardized and differ between institutions.

37.2.2.3   Treatment

Insurance restrictions: four times before and two times after transplantation

Modality: Same as in ABO incompatible transplantation

Actual frequency: Same as in ABO incompatible transplantation

Therapeutic target: Eliminating anti-donor specific HLA antibody to undetectable levels is ideal but no consensus exists on the target level.

37.3   Apheresis After Transplantation

37.3.1   Antibody Mediated Rejection

37.3.1.1   Target of Elimination and Pathophysiology

Target: Mainly IgG anti-donor specific HLA antibody or anti-A or -B IgG, IgM antibody

Pathophysiology: Antigen–antibody reaction due to anti donor specific HLA antibody or anti-A, -B antibody directed at donor kidney.

37.3.1.2   Therapeutic Effect

Treatment is based on intensifying immunosuppression by the elimination of antibodies with therapeutic apheresis. The simultaneous use of apheresis, immunosuppressants, and intravenous immunoglobulins (IVIG) have been shown to effectively treat antibody mediated rejection. However, renal survival after hyperacute rejection is extremely poor.

37.3.1.3 Treatment

Insurance restrictions: There is no indication for apheresis after transplantation for antibody mediated rejection.

Modality: Same as in ABO-incompatible transplantation

Actual frequency: Varies on the response and severity but many institutions implement two three sessions or more.

Therapeutic target: Anti-donor specific HLA antibody and anti-A or -B antibody may be absorbed by the donated kidney and show fairly low levels of antibody titers shortly after transplantation. Therefore, antibody titers may not reflect the activity of rejection. Furthermore, antibodies other than anti-donor specific HLA antibodies have been reported to cause antibody related rejection, which further complicates the diagnosis. The diagnosis of antibody related rejection therefore may rely on the synthetic judgment of urinary output, rising serum creatinine levels, and pre-transplant antibody titer shortly after transplantation. A biopsy is normally undertaken to confirm the diagnosis. In cases of ABO-incompatible transplantation, anti-A or -B titers increasing 2 weeks after transplantation may not reflect or induce antibody mediated rejection due to the mechanism of accommodation. However, anti-A or -B titers increasing rapidly within 2 weeks may be treated with apheresis as prophylaxis for rejection. Recent reports show poor long-term renal prognosis in recipients with high anti-HLA antibodies after transplantation [4], which suggests the need for further studies on the role of immunosuppression and apheresis.

37.3.2 Renal Disease Other than Antibody Mediated Rejection

Recurrence of focal segmental glomerulosclerosis (FSGS) after kidney transplantation is quite frequent (20–50 %) and treatment with apheresis, a strategy not unique to transplant patients, may be suggested. Recurrence of FSGS is known to affect renal survival (renal loss after FSGS recurrence is

13–20 %) [5]. Apheresis treatment of FSGS recurrence in kidney transplant patients is done in the same way as in non-transplant FSGS.

37.4 Therapies Other than Apheresis

37.4.1 Immunosuppression Before Kidney Transplantation

Immunosuppression directed against T cells and B cells is initiated before transplantation in living related kidney transplantation. Sufficient immunosuppression is especially needed in patients with high anti-A or -B titers in ABO incompatible transplantation, high anti-donor specific HLA antibody titers, and/or high rebound in titers after apheresis. The most frequently used immunosuppression regimen consists of calcineurin inhibitors, anti-metabolites, steroids, and anti-CD20 monoclonal antibodies (basiliximab). In ABO-incompatible transplantation, splenectomy is done adjunctively for additional B cell depletion. However, recent studies show favorable outcome with rituximab (anti-CD20 antibody) use as an alternative to splenectomy [6] and is now widely used as a standard protocol in most institutes. Unfortunately, use of rituximab in ABO-incompatible transplantation is still not covered by insurance in Japan which limits its use in some institutions.

37.4.2 Immunosuppression After Kidney Transplantation

In cases of uncontrollable antibody mediated rejection even after the sufficient use of immunosuppressants, splenectomy, and rituximab, IVIG administration may be required. If kidney function is unfortunately lost, transplant nephrectomy may be necessary in cases of poor general status (such as disseminated intravascular coagulation) and enlarged kidney, leading to risk of kidney rupture.

Notes: ABO-Incompatible Transplantation

Specific examples are (1) type A to B or O; (2) type B to A or O; (3) type AB to A, B, or O.

Evaluation of anti-donor specific HLA antibody

Tissue typing tests are obligatory. A commonly used technique is the complement dependent cytotoxicity (CDC) test in which complement activation triggered by the recipient antibody binding on the surface of the donor antigen-expressing lymphocytes may lyse the cells. The advantage of this test is that it can detect the strength of cytotoxic effect, but its sensitivity is low. Recently, the more sensitive flow cytometric crossmatch (FCMX) test is used to detect antigen–antibody reactions between the donor lymphocytes and recipient serum. Other tests using flow cytometry and Luminex technology are available for detecting specific HLAs. Secondary transplantation, history of blood transfusion, and pregnancy (especially when the recipient has borne the child of the donor) are well known risks of anti-HLA antibody production.

Definition of Antibody Mediated Rejection

Pathological definitions of T cell or antibody mediated rejection are defined in the Banff 07 classification of renal allograft pathology. Antibody mediated rejection is defined as the existence of anti-donor specific HLA antibodies and C4d staining at the peritubular capillaries and morphologic evidence of tissue injury in the tubules (ATN-like inflammation), glomerulus (inflammation and/or thrombosis), or arteries (arteritis) [7].

References

1. Takahashi K (2008) ABO-incompatible kidney transplantation: update. Nihon Jinzo Gakkaishi 50(7):880–886
2. Nishi S (2009) Jin-ishoku no subete. Medical View co Ltd, Tokyo, pp 80–81

3. Tanabe K (2006) Jin-ishoku no shinnpo wagakunino genjyou to kongo no tenbou. Tokyo igakusha, Tokyo, pp 101–110
4. Lee P, Zhu L, Terasaki PI et al (2009) Transplantation 88(4): 568–574
5. Choy B, Chan T, Lai K (2006) Am J Transplant 6(11):2535–2542
6. Saito K, Nakagawa Y, Suwa M et al (2006) Xenotransplantation 13(2):111–117
7. Solez K, Colvin R, Racusen L et al (2007) Am J Transplant 7(3): 518–526

Chapter 38
Peripheral Blood Stem Cell Transplantation

Naoko Watanabe-Okochi

Main Points
- CD34 positive hematopoietic stem cells are mobilized from bone marrow to peripheral blood by G-CSF administration, and collected using a blood cell separator that uses a centrifuge to separate mononuclear cells.

38.1 Peripheral Blood Stem Cell Transplantation

Peripheral blood stem cell transplantation (PBSCT) is an indispensable treatment option for progressive malignant diseases. Autologous PBSCT is usually performed on patients with malignant disease without residual malignant cells in

N. Watanabe-Okochi (✉)
Department of transfusion, University Hospital, The University of Tokyo,
7-3-1 Hongo, Bunkyo-ku, Tokyo 113-8655, Japan
e-mail: nokochiwatanabe-tky@umin.ac.jp

E. Noiri and N. Hanafusa (eds.), *The Concise Manual of Apheresis Therapy*, DOI 10.1007/978-4-431-54412-8_38,
© Springer Japan 2014

bone marrow. Allogeneic PBSCT is usually performed on patients with progressive hematological malignancies. PBSCs have advantages in terms of early engraftment compared with other transplantable sources such as bone marrow cells and cord blood cells, and PBSCT is predominantly performed in Western countries.

38.2   Peripheral Blood Stem Cell Harvest (PBSCH)

38.2.1   Susceptible Diseases and Donors

38.2.1.1   Target Cells of Harvest

The target cells for harvest in PBSCT are peripheral blood CD34 positive hematopoietic stem cells.

38.2.1.2   Susceptible Disease for Auto PBSCH

Diseases that are indications for autologous PBSCT are acute promyelocytic leukemia, malignant lymphoma, multiple myeloma, germ cell tumor, neuroblastoma, small cell carcinoma, et al without bone marrow invasion.

38.2.1.3   Donor Eligibility

High dose granulocyte-colony stimulating factor (G-CSF) administration is performed to healthy donors to collect CD34 positive peripheral blood stem cells. For the donor's safety, screening and the exclusion of those who risk serious adverse events associated with G-CSF administration is important. Accordingly, the Japan Society of Transfusion Medicine and Cell Therapy (JSTMCT) and the Japan Society for Hematopoietic Cell Transplantation (JSHCT)

TABLE 38.1 Disqualification criteria for donor blood cell donation (quoted from guideline [1])

Donors who have risks associated with G-CSF administration
• Allergic reaction to G-CSF
• History and/or risk of thrombosis: hypertension, coronary disease, diabetes, hyperlipidemia
• Splenomegaly
• Suspect of myeloproliferative disorder: leukocytosis, thrombocytosis
• History of interstitial pneumonia
• History of malignant disease
• Autoimmune disorder
• Pregnancy
• Cardiovascular disease, pulmonary disease, renal disorder under medical treatment
• Hepatic dysfunction
• Neurological disorder

proposed guidelines for donor selection (Table 38.1). These also recommend selecting donors from 10 to 65 years old and require the approval of the ethics board in each facility, if said donors are under 10 or over 65 years of age [1].

Peripheral blood stem cells have the advantage of early engraftment compared with other transplantable sources such as bone marrow cells and cord blood cells, and PBSCH does not require general anesthesia unlike bone marrow cell donation. However, this process risks adverse effects associated with G-CSF administration for healthy donors and high rates of serious chronic graft versus host disease (GVHD) for recipients. It is still undecided which is safer to use as hematopoietic stem cell sources, and is therefore controversial.

38.2.2   PBSC Mobilization

38.2.2.1   G-CSF Administration

Donors receive G-CSF for 3–4 days prior to the start of apheresis. A total of 400 mg/m^2 per day G-CSF (Filgrastim) and 10 mg/kg per day G-CSF (lenograstim) are applicable to medical insurance in Japan. The twice daily subcutaneous injection is more efficient in mobilizing PBSC in normal donors than is a single injection [2, 3]. The twice daily subcutaneous injection requires fewer apheresis procedures without increasing toxicity. The G-CSF injection is continued if the target CD34+ cell yield is not achieved. After G-CSF administration, the complete blood count (CBC) and the white blood cell (WBC) fraction should be examined. If WBC exceeds 50,000 cells/μL, the G-CSF dose should be reduced. If it exceeds 75,000 cells/μL, the G-CSF injections should cease.

38.2.2.2   Optimal Timing of PBSCH

The peak of CD34+ cell mobilization is observed on day 5 after G-CSF administration, then CD34+ cell counts decrease after day 7, and continuous administration is less effective [4]. Therefore apheresis usually starts from day 4 or 5. As a reduction in the CD34+ cell count occurs at 1–2 h after G-CSF administration and recovers to baseline within 3–4 h, G-CSF should be given 4 h prior to stem cell collection [5].

In autologous PBSCH, it is difficult to optimize the CD34+ cell collection timing because the recovery speed of WBCs after chemotherapy depends on the primary disease treatment and individual bone marrow state. The number of CD34+ cells in peripheral blood is a guide to the optimal timing to harvest peripheral blood stem cells. The minimum number of CD34+ cells in PB to collect 1.5×10^6/kg CD34+ cells is over 15 CD34+ cells/μL [6]. However, CD34+ cell count requires specific equipment and several hours to obtain results. Therefore, the measurement of peripheral blood

CD34+ cells prior to just before the apheresis is not available in all facilities. Facilities which cannot utilize peripheral CD34+ cell count as a predictive factor need to base on other predictive values. For examples, increase of monocyte rates, reticulocyte numbers, and LDH values are used as predictive factors for the CD34+ cell yield. When there is a sharp increase in WBC compared with that of the previous day (for example, 500 to 2,500/μL), there is a possibility of achieving sufficient CD34+ cells even if the total WBC is lower than 2,500/μL. Hematopoietic progenitor cell (HPC) quantification is also used to predict the timing of CD34+ cell mobilization [7]. Over 25 HPC cells/μL is recommended for starting PBSC collection.

38.2.2.3   Poor Mobilization

PBSC mobilization failure occurs in some donors and patients (poor mobilization). Although there is no predictive factor for poor mobilization at this point, poor mobilizers are frequently elderly. It is important to inform all related patients of the possibility of stem cell source change from PBSC to BM due to insufficient CD34+ cell yields.

38.2.3   Apheresis

38.2.3.1   Blood Access

Blood access is established via either side of two antecubital veins by 17- to 19-gauge crump catheters for both the inlet and return lines. Complete disinfection around the puncture of a vein is important to minimize the risk of infection. Binding the inlet side arms and asking the patient to clasp a tennis ball are useful to maintain the desired blood flow rate. When blood access is difficult, this can be rectified by inserting a double lumen catheter to a central vein for the inlet and return lines.

38.2.3.2   Mononuclear Cell Isolation

A PBSCH is a procedure involving the isolation and collection of mononuclear cells from the peripheral blood using a centrifuge method. The collected mononuclear cells include CD34+ hematopoietic stem cells, monocytes, lymphocytes, and erythroblasts. When the hematocrit value is lower than 25 %, it is difficult to collect mononuclear cells because of an insufficient red blood cell layer under the mononuclear cell layer. Therefore, red blood cell transfusion should be considered when hematocrit value is lower than 30 % or hemoglobin level is lower than 9 g/dL. Processing blood volume is determined ranging from 150–250 mL/kg, or twice to three times the total blood volume. Blood flow is determined ranging from body weight (kg) milliliters per minute to 70 mL per minute. When the processed blood volume has achieved the desired value, blood should be sampled, and the needles removed from the veins. Because a acid citrate dextrose solution is used as an anticoagulant, arrest of bleeding must be confirmed before the patient leaves the apheresis room. A progress note during apheresis should be written and kept. At 1–2 weeks after the apheresis, the donor's (or the patient's) blood cell count and spleen size should finally be confirmed as having returned to normal values.

38.2.3.3   The Minimum Amount of CD34 Positive Cells

The dose of CD34+ cells should be evaluated in conformity with the guideline of the International Society of Hematotherapy and Graft Engineering (ISHAGE) [8]. The minimum amount of CD34+ cells are 1.0×10^6 cells/kg recipient body weight for auto PBSCT and 2.0×10^6/kg for allo PBSCT, respectively. For tandem auto transplantation and HLA mismatch allo PBSCT, the targeted CD34 positive cell yield needs to exceed 3.0×10^6/kg.

38.2.3.4   Preservation of Hematopoietic Stem Cells

Use a clean bench for cell processing with more than one person. Make a cell protective reagent using CP1 (mixture of hydroxyethyl starch: HES and Dimethylsulfoxide: DMSO) and 4 % albumin. Adjust the cell concentration to less than 5.0×10^7 cells/mL in the cell protective reagent. Transfer the collected cells from a collection bag to a frozen bag, and mix with the cell protective reagent slowly. Take a sampling of approximately 1 mL for retrospective analysis. Keep the frozen bag in a specific protector to freeze in −80 °C for 24 h, then transfer the protector to a liquid nitrogen tank and keep at −196 °C. Write note freezing method such as cell protective reagent, cell concentration, positive rates of CD34 and CD3.

38.2.4   Adverse Events

38.2.4.1   Hypocalcaemia

Anticoagulant citrate dextrose solution, Solution A, (ACD-A) is used as an anticoagulant in the extracorporeal blood processing for PBSCH. As citrate-based anticoagulants prevent the coagulation of blood by chelating ionized calcium, hypocalcaemia is the most frequent adverse effect during PBSCH. Continuous administration of calcium gluconate during apheresis is recommended. Otherwise, when hypocalcaemia occurs, administer calcium gluconate slowly.

38.2.4.2   Thrombocytopenia

Platelets are lost during apheresis. Therefore, a platelet concentration 50,000/µL is needed before starting apheresis. Upon completion of apheresis, the peripheral blood cell count should be checked.

38.2.4.3   Others

Dizziness, nausea, vomiting, vaso-vagal reflex (VVR) and temporary hypovolemic symptoms can occur. Consequently, monitoring ECG and blood pressure and careful observation by an apheresis specialist are important.

38.2.5   Column

An apheresis usually takes 3–4 h and subjects may feel tired and experience some discomfort during the procedure from the double insertion of needles. Therefore, comfortable environments should be prepared for subjects, for example, exclusive space, exclusive beds, blankets, TV, and music.

References

1. Guideline for peripheral blood stem cell mobilization and collection from healthy donors for allogeneic peripheral blood stem cell transplantation. The Japan Society for hematopoietic cell transplantation. The Japan Society of transfusion medicine and cell therapy (a revised edition version 3), 21 April 2003
2. Lee V, Li CK, Shing MM et al (2000) Single vs twice daily G-CSF dose for peripheral blood stem cells harvest in normal donors and children with non-malignant diseases. Bone Marrow Transplant 25:931–935
3. Kröger N, Renges H, Krüger W et al (2000) A randomized comparison of once versus twice daily recombinant human granulocyte colony-stimulating factor (filgrastim) for stem cell mobilization in healthy donors for allogeneic transplantation. Br J Haematol 111:761–765
4. Stroncek DF, Clay ME, Petzoldt ML et al (1996) Treatment of normal individuals with granulocyte-colony-stimulating factor: donor experiences and the effects on peripheral blood CD34+ cell counts and on the collection of peripheral blood stem cells. Transfusion 36:601–610

5. Watts MJ, Addison I, Ings SJ et al (1998) Optimal timing for collection of PBPC after glycosylated G-CSF administration. Bone Marrow Transplant 21:365–368
6. Basquiera AL, Abichain P, Damonte JC et al (2006) The number of CD34(+) cells in peripheral blood as a predictor of the CD34(+) yield in patients going to autologous stem cell transplantation. J Clin Apher 21:92–5
7. Kawakami K, Abe Y, Imataki O et al (2006) Determining the time of harvesting peripheral blood stem cells using the HPC, for monitoring hematopoietic progenitor cells, of the automated hematology analyzer XE-2100. Sysmex J 29:39–45
8. Sutherland DR, Anderson L, Keeney M, Nayar R, Chin-Yee I (1996) The ISHAGE guidelines for CD34+ cell determination by flow cytometry. International Society of Hematotherapy and Graft Engineering. J Hematother 5:213–26

Part VII
Pediatric Apheresis

Chapter 39
Apheresis in Children

Motoshi Hattori

Main Points

- It has become possible to perform apheresis in small children owing to the development and clinical application of specialized blood purification devices and equipment, such as vascular catheters for small children and small-volume extracorporeal circuits and modules.

- Technical considerations include ensuring vascular access, reducing extracorporeal volume, preventing hypothermia, and providing proper anti-coagulant treatment.

M. Hattori (✉)
Department of Pediatric Nephrology, Tokyo Women's Medical University,
School of Medicine, 8-1 Kawada-cho, Shinjuku-ku, Tokyo 162-8666, Japan
e-mail: hattori@kc.twmu.ac.jp

E. Noiri and N. Hanafusa (eds.), *The Concise Manual*
of Apheresis Therapy, DOI 10.1007/978-4-431-54412-8_39,
© Springer Japan 2014

39.1   Indications for Therapeutic Apheresis in Children

Diseases indicated for apheresis are the same for both pediatric and adult patients. For example, plasma exchange (PE) therapy is provided for fulminant hepatitis, focal segmental glomerulosclerosis (FSGS), and thrombotic microangiopathy; plasma adsorption (PA) therapy for endotoxemia and gram-negative bacterial infection; and leukocytapheresis for ulcerative colitis. These procedures are all covered by regular health insurance in Japan.

Moreover, the medical fee revision in 2012 introduced health insurance coverage for PE therapy in patients with Kawasaki disease not responding to an intravenous immunoglobulin, steroid therapy, or neutrophil elastase inhibitor in Japan.

Although there are a variety of causes for hemolytic uremic syndrome (HUS), approximately 90 % of pediatric HUS cases are caused by Shiga toxin (also known as verotoxin)-producing *Escherichia coli* (STEC) infection, for which apheresis is not indicated [1, 2]. In contrast, apheresis is indicated for atypical HUS (aHUS) caused by abnormalities in complement regulatory proteins [1, 2] (Table 39.1).

39.2   Technical Considerations

39.2.1   Vascular Access

The double-lumen central venous catheters are used to secure vascular access (VA) in pediatric apheresis. Although several types of pediatric catheters are available on the market, the Baby-Flow catheter (6 Fr) from Unitika (Tokyo, Japan) has the narrowest diameter suitable for use in small children weighing over 3 kg [3]. The Tornado-Flow double-lumen catheter with an end-hole (7 Fr) (Covidien

TABLE 39.1 Etiology of HUS and indication for apheresis

Etiology	Indication
STEC	No
CFH	Yes
CHI	Yes
CFH autoantobody	Yes
MCP	No
CFB	Yes
C3 convertase	Yes
Thrombomodulin	Yes

STEC Shiga toxin-producing *Escherichia coli*, *CFH* complement factor H, *CHI* complement factor I, *MCP* membrane co-factor protein, *CFB* complement factor B, *HUS* hemolytic uremic syndrome

Japan, Tokyo, Japan) is also useful because it reduces the pressure of returning blood [3]. Catheters 10 Fr or larger can be used in children weighing over 20 kg [3]. The length, gage, and positioning of the tip of the catheter will depend on the child's size.

39.2.2 Extracorporeal Volume (ECV) and Devices

When performing apheresis in small children, technicians may find it easier and safer to use a special device with a small volume circuit (Table 39.2) [4]. Reducing the ECV with the use of a small-volume extracorporeal circuit and module is essential in pediatric apheresis.

Extracorporeal circuits and modules are selected so that ECV remains at less than 10 % of the total blood volume

TABLE 39.2 Small-volume systems in pediatric apheresis

Manufacturer	System	Circuit line	PV (mL)	Arterial chamber
Asahi Kasei Medical	ACH-10	PT-400NLl	79.5	Yes
	Plasauto iQ21	PE-P21C	44.7	No
	PlasautoS	CRRT-PSGAL	46	No
Toray Medical	TR-55X	U-520SH	43	No
		U-525MC	39	Yes
Kawasumi	KM-8900a	HF277	44	Yes
Laboratories	KM-9000	K-PE-90PEP	60	Yes

PV priming volume

(TBV) (the weight-based estimated TBV is 70–75 mL/kg) [4]. However, this is not applicable in newborns and infants, and therefore it is necessary to prime the circuit with blood products before starting apheresis. When patients are receiving vasopressor agents, the dosage of these agents should be increased temporarily as a countermeasure to the dilution of their blood concentrations [4].

Plasmaflo (OP-02W) manufactured by Asahi Kasei Medical (Tokyo, Japan) is the only small-volume plasma separator available on the market in Japan. With this membrane, the ECV, including plasma side, during single PE is slightly less than 60 mL [4].

Double filtration plasmapheresis (DFPP) and PA therapies in small children have been conventionally considered difficult in terms of ECV. However, their application has recently been increasing because of the efforts made by individual manufacturers to develop small-volume systems, including extracorporeal blood circuits. For example, the Lipid Apheresis Machine MA-03 by Kaneka (Tokyo, Japan) used in a low-density lipoprotein apheresis (LA-15 manufactured by Kaneka) is equipped with a removable heating element, which reduces ECV by 25 mL, making the final ECV on both sides 290 mL (OP-02W, 25 mL; LA-15, 140 mL; circuit line, 125 mL) [4].

A greater number of membrane sizes and materials are now available for continuous renal replacement therapy. A membrane area of 0.1 m^2 is on the market, and for membranes with an area of 0.3 m^2, there are three different materials to choose from [4].

39.2.3   Hypothermia

Children and adults experience some degree of hypothermia during apheresis procedures because of the cooling of blood in the extracorporeal circuit. This side effect is more pronounced in children as the ECV to patient body surface area is higher than that for adults [5]. Small children are more susceptible to hypothermia because of larger ventilation volume/minute per body weight, smaller subcutaneous fat amount, and higher percutaneous water transpiration due to their thin and immature skin [4].

A blood warmer is incorporated into the return line in pediatric apheresis procedures [5]. In addition, using an infant warmer and/or wrapping the circuit with aluminum foil are helpful to prevent hypothermia [4].

39.2.4   Anticoagulation

Anticoagulation to prevent clotting in the extracorporeal circuit is essential for successful execution of apheresis. Unfractionated heparin or nafamostat mesylate (Torii, Tokyo, Japan) in patients with a high risk of bleeding has been used widely as an anti-coagulant in Japan [4]. Although low-molecular-weight heparin is also used in adults in Japan, its use in children is rare because of the difficulty of bedside monitoring [4].

When blood flow rate (Q_B) is less than 20–30 mL/min, it takes a long time for the blood entering the circuit to be returned to the body, and blood may be retained in the drip chamber. Therefore, as a precautionary measure, it is sometimes necessary to increase the dose by a maximum of 1.5 times the normal dose while monitoring the activated coagulation time (ACT) of the whole blood. ACT is used in dose monitoring because it can be easily measured at the bedside. The Hemochron Jr. Signature Plus device (ITC, Edison, USA) allows the measurement of ACT from a single drop (approximately 0.2 mL) of blood [4].

39.3   Practice of PE Therapy

39.3.1   Replacement Fluid

Fresh frozen plasma (FFP) is used as a replacement fluid in PE to supplement coagulation factors and approximately 100–150 mL/kg per session of FFP are replaced in pediatric patients with fulminant hepatitis [4]. In PE for patients with post-transplant recurrence of FSGS, approximately 50–60 mL/kg per session of human albumin solutions are replaced and generally 70 % of plasma IgG was removed per one session [4].

39.3.2   Actual Treatment Conditions

These are simple objectives that we use to treat children weighing approximately 10 kg.

Q_B is set at 20–30 mL/m (2–3 mL/m per kg). There is no need to increase Q_B unless necessary because an increase in Q_B does not result in an improved treatment efficacy. It is also not advantageous to reduce Q_B too much because it would prolong the circuit transit time. The plasma flow rate (Q_p) is set at 20 % of Q_B at most, and an increase in the transmembrane pressure difference needs to be carefully monitored [4].

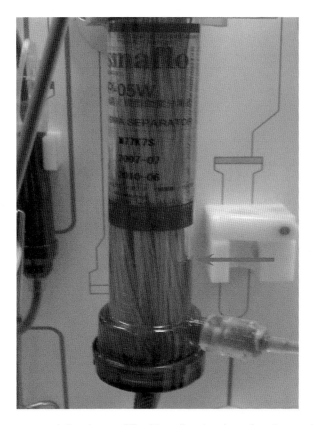

FIGURE 39.1 Adjustment of liquid surface level on the plasma side of a plasma separator. By lowering the liquid surface level on the plasma side in the plasma separator to 1/4th of the total volume (*arrow*), a reduction of the extracorporeal volume can be achieved

In addition, for the purpose of reducing ECV, we lower the liquid surface level on the plasma side in the plasma separator to 1/4th of the total volume (Fig. 39.1).

Lastly, a diagram of the serial and parallel circuit and treatment conditions that we use for concurrent slow PE and continuous hemodiafiltration (CHDF) are presented in Fig. 39.2.

410   M. Hattori

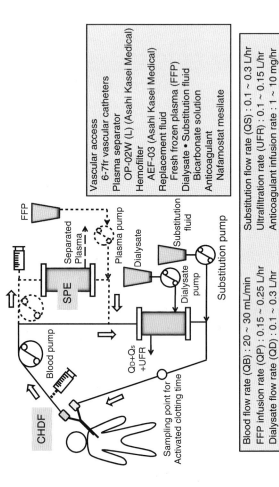

FIGURE 39.2 Diagram of the serial and parallel circuit of concurrent slow plasma exchange (SPE) and continuous hemodiafiltration (CHDF). Devices and treatment conditions that we use to treat children weighing approximately 10 kg are also presented

References

1. Wong ECC, Balogun RA (2012) Therapeutic apheresis in pediatrics: technique adjustments, indications and nonindications, a plasma exchange focus. J Clin Apheresis 27:132–137
2. Waters AM, Licht C (2011) A HUS caused by complement deregulation: new therapies on the horizon. Pediatr Nephrol 26:41–54
3. Soma I, Hattori M (2011) Vascular access for pediatric patients. Rinsho-Touseki 27:839–848 (in Japanese)
4. Soma I, Hattori M (2010) Blood purification in children. In: Apheresis manual revised 3 version. Japanese Society for Apheresis, Syujunsya, pp 184–191 (in Japanese)
5. Goldstein SL (2012) Therapeutic apheresis in children: special considerations. Semin Dial 25:165–170

Index

E. Noiri and N. Hanafusa (eds.), *The Concise Manual of Apheresis Therapy*, DOI 10.1007/978-4-431-54412-8,
© Springer Japan 2014

414   Index